Electrocardiography
Pocket Handbook

Electrocardiography Pocket Handbook

Derek J. Rowlands

Consultant Cardiologist
Manchester Royal Infirmary
Hon. Lecturer in Cardiology
University of Manchester, UK

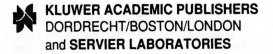

KLUWER ACADEMIC PUBLISHERS
DORDRECHT/BOSTON/LONDON
and **SERVIER LABORATORIES**

Thanks are due to ICI Pharmaceuticals for permission to adapt certain diagrams from the publication **Understanding the Electrocardiogram** by Dr D.J. Rowlands (© Imperial Chemical Industries 1987)

Distributors

for the United States and Canada:
Kluwer Academic Publishers, PO Box 358, Accord Station, Hingham, MA 02018-0358, USA

for all other countries:
Kluwer Academic Publishers Group, Distribution Center, PO Box 322, 3300 AH Dordrecht, The Netherlands

A catalogue record for this book is available from the British Library

ISBN 0-7923-8805-4

Copyright

Co-published in the United Kingdom by Kluwer Academic Publishers, PO Box 55, Lancaster, UK and Servier Laboratories. Kluwer Academic Publishers BV incorporates the publishing programmes of D. Reidel, Martinus Nijhoff, Dr W. Junk and MTP Press

Designed and Typeset by Graham C. Agnew, Over Kellet, Lancashire. Printed and bound in Great Britain by Pindar Graphics, Preston.

Contents

Foreword   9

1 The Normal ECG   10

What is an electrocardiogram?   11

ECG leads   13
Bibipolar recordings   13
Unipolar leads   13
Unipolar limb leads   14
Unipolar precordial leads   16
Electrode position   17
The technique of recording   18
The electrocardiographic tracing   18
A typical recording   19

Analysis of the different elements in the
electrocardiogram   21

The P wave   21
The P-R interval   23
The QRS complex   25
QRS terminology   25
QRS dimensions   26
The pathological QRS complex   27
Intrinsic and intrinsicoid deflections   28
The S-T interval   29
The T wave   31
The U wave   32

The electrical axis   33

Determination of the electrical axis   36

The significance of the axis   42

2 The Pathological ECG 43

Electrical alterations in hypertrophy of muscle or enlargement of the chambers 44

The atrial hypertrophies 44

Left atrial hypertrophy 44
Right atrial hypertrophy 46
Right atrial hypertrophy, accompanied by a right ventricular hypertrophy 47
Bi-atrial hypertrophy 48

The ventricular hypertrophies 51

Left ventricular hypertrophy 51
Left ventricular hypertrophy (systolic overload) 54
Left ventricular hypertrophy (diastolic overload) 56
Right ventricular hypertrophy 58
Biventricular hypertrophy 60

Electrical abnormalities in disease of the coronary circulation 63

Myocardial infarction 63

Alteration of the QRS 64
Alteration of the S–T 63

Schematic representation of the evolution of the electrical changes in myocardial infarction 68

ECG localization of infarctions 69

Extensive anterior myocardial infarction 70
Antero-septal myocardial infarction 72
Antero-lateral myocardial infarction 74
Inferior myocardial infarction 76

Acute and chronic coronary insufficiency 78

Antero-lateral sub-endocardial ischaemic lesion 79
Extensive sub-epicardial anterior myocardial ischaemia 80

Electrical disturbances in the disorders of conduction and activation 82

The pathway of depolarization in the cardiac muscle 83

At the level of the sino-atrial (SA) node 84

Normal and abnormal rhythm initiated at the SA node   84
Sinus tachycardia and bradycardia   85
Sinus arrhythmias, sinus arrest, sino-atrial block
and AV nodal escape   88

Ectopic rhythms at the level of the atrial myocardium   92

Atrial tachycardia   93
Atrial flutter and fibrillation   94

Ectopic rhythms at the level of the atrio-ventricular junction
(ie the low right atrium or the atrio-ventricular node)   97

Paroxysmal supraventricular tachycardia   98

Escape rhythms at the level of the atrio-ventricular node   104

Nodal rhythm   106

Conduction disturbance at the level of the His
bundle or the atrio-ventricular node   111

The atrio-ventricular block (heart block)   112
First degree incomplete heart block   112
Second degree atrio-ventricular block   114
Third degree atrio-ventricular block (complete heart block)   118

At the level of the branches of the bundle of His,
ie Bundle Branch Block   120

Complete bundle branch blocks   121
Complete left bundle branch block   121
Complete right bundle branch block   125
Incomplete RBBB and incomplete LBBB   127

Ventricular pre-excitation   128

At the level of the ventricular myocardium   132

Ventricular extrasystoles   140
Bigeminal ventricular extrasystoles   142
Multiple and polymorphic ventricular extrasystoles   143

Miscellaneous abnormalities (pericardial, metabolism,
endocrine and drug-induced)   144

Acute pericarditis   144
ECG in abnormal metabolic states   146

Bibliography   154

Foreword

It is over 100 years since the first human ECG was recorded by A.D. Waller in 1887. Waller wrote that he did not imagine that electrocardiography was likely to find extensive use in hospitals but Einthoven, in Holland, and Thomas Lewis, in England, pioneered the clinical application of electrocardiography. The 12-lead ECG is now an essential part of any cardiac assessment. Over 100 million 12-lead ECGs are now recorded annually worldwide and the importance of the electrocardiogram in clinical practice has not diminished with the development of numerous other investigative and imaging techniques. Each new generation of doctors needs to acquire an understanding of the ECG.

The original "Notes on Electrocardiography" was written many years ago, by a French doctor. His name is unknown but his initials were B.R. My brief was to read the original manuscript, correct any perceived errors and bring the concepts up to date, wherever relevant. This was not an easy task. One was tempted either to leave the manuscript alone or to alter it completely. In the event, I chose to adhere to the original layout (chapter headings and order) and to use the original illustrations wherever possible. I would not have chosen to deal with things in the order chosen by B.R. but this approach does have merit. The end result inevitably involves inhomogeneities. The reader will probably have little difficulty in recognising those parts which I have completely re-written and the illustrations and text which are completely new. Hopefully, the fact that one can "see the join" should not detract from the usefulness of this pocket-sized introduction to electrocardiography.

I am happy to acknowledge the fundamental work done by B.R., who was clearly an experienced teacher of electrocardiography. I hope that he would take a tolerant view of my own contribution and that the modern reader will find that this booklet provides a relatively painless introduction to the important and complex subject of clinical electrocardiography.

D.J. Rowlands

What is an electrocardiogram?

It is an electrical recording of the potentials called the action potentials which occur prior to contraction of cardiac muscle.

All muscle produces electrical activity in relation to contraction and the heart is not an exception to this rule.

Each living cell is polarized and if such a cell is excited, it enters a state of physical activity divided into two phases, rapid depolarization and then a period of slow repolarization. In the course of excitation of a cell or a muscle, one can record a potential change in only one direction – a monophasic response.

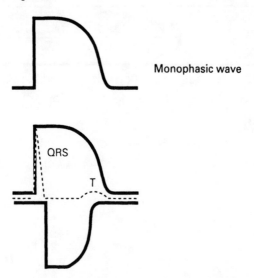

Monophasic wave

The surface ECG is the resultant of very many myocardial cells, each producing its own action potential. The times of initiation, the directions of travel and the durations of the action potentials are not all the same.

The surface ECG has two main recognizable waves, resulting from the action potential in the ventricular myocardium, the QRS and the T wave. The way in which varied action potentials of individual cells gives rise to the QRS and T wave can be understood from a consideration of two monophasic action potentials of opposite sign (ie travelling in opposite directions). If the second action potential starts marginally after the first and if the duration action potential of the second cell is significantly less than that of the first, then upright deflections will result at the beginning and at the end of the action potential (QRS and T wave).

Two types of recording of the ECG are used: bipolar and
unipolar.

Bipolar recordings

Two electrodes are put on the surface of the body and the
electrical activity of the heart produces an electrical potential
between them. Thus both leads contribute to the resulting
record.

Since Einthoven, three bipolar leads have always been
recorded, known as the "standard leads". The electrodes are
strapped to both wrists and to the left ankle.

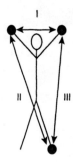

Lead I between right and left arms
Lead II between right arm and left leg
Lead III between left arm and left leg

Standard bipolar leads and Einthoven triangle

Unipolar leads

Here, two electrodes are used, but one of them remains at zero
potential and the other electrode is used to measure change in
potential produced in the limbs (unipolar limb aVR, aVL, aVF)
or at different points over the precordium and chest
(precordial leads V_1 to V_6). The zero electrode is achieved by
connecting all three limb leads together.

Unipolar limb leads

Three unipolar leads record the difference in potential existing between the zero reference electrode and the limb potential.

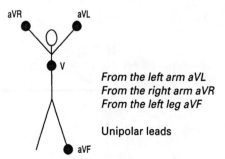

From the left arm aVL
From the right arm aVR
From the left leg aVF

Unipolar leads

The potential differences coming from the heart are represented by a vector, V, whose origin is at the centre of the Einthoven triangle and whose projection on each of three sides of the triangle produces the corresponding standard leads, I, II and III.

One can imagine the three standard leads as the sides of a triangle with the heart in the centre.

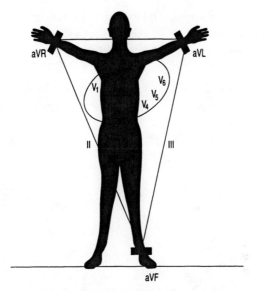

The tracings obtained in these three leads are the projections on each side of the triangle of the electrical potentials resulting from cardiac excitation.

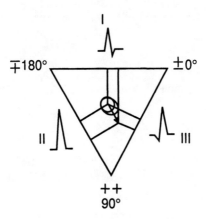

An alternative way of thinking about the limb leads is to consider them as directions (rather than sides or apices of a triangle). In this case, the arrangement is:

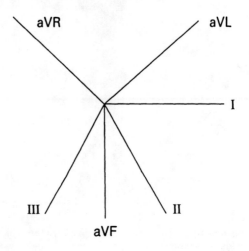

Unipolar precordial leads

The six leads most frequently used are V_1, V_2, V_3, V_4, V_5, V_6, and the diagram opposite shows the position of the precordial electrodes.

• Sometimes one uses:

V_3R and V_4R symmetrical with V_3, V_4, but to the right of the sternum.

The complementary leads V_7, V_8.

• The oesophageal lead is only of historic interest.

Electrode position

1) Frontal view
Standard and unipolar limb leads

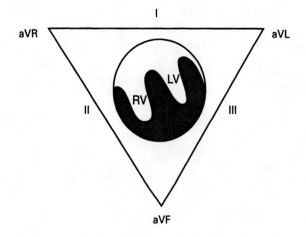

2) Horizontal plan
Precordial leads

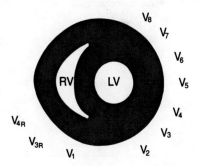

17

The technique of recording

The recording paper usually has horizontal and vertical markings.

a) The horizontal lines show the amplitude – they are spaced 1 mm apart and every fifth line is darker than the others. One centimetre corresponds to one millivolt.

b) The vertical lines show the time intervals. Again, every fifth line is darker. Each small space represents 0.04 sec and each larger 0.2 sec.

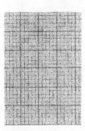

The electrocardiographic tracing

Whatever the lead, the tracing is composed of a number of fundamental components. During the resting period, the tracing is said to be at the isoelectric level.

With each cardiac contraction are drawn:

- A first deflection, the P wave of small amplitude, corresponding to atrial contraction.

- A latent period during atrio-ventricular conduction.
- The ventricular complex, composed of rapid, large deflections of short duration, the first often downwards, Q, the second upwards, R, and a third, downward deflection, S. Each of these may be of great or small amplitude.
- The ventricular complex also has a slow T wave, usually upwards, possibly followed by a U wave (best seen in lead II). The Q-T interval measures the duration of ventricular excitation.
- The isoelectric line is seen during the T-P interval.

A typical recording

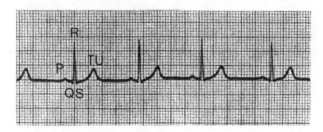

P   = atrial depolarization
PR   = atrio-ventricular conduction
QRS = rapid ventricular depolarization (qRs)
T   = slow ventricular repolarization wave
U   = follows T wave and may or may not be visible
ST   = normally isoelectric
QT   = length of the ventricular complex

Length of the different components in the tracing:
P   = less than 0.1 sec
PR   = 0.12-0.20 sec
QRS < 0.12 sec usually 0.05-0.08 sec
QT   = 0.38-0.40 sec

In the unipolar leads:

• The deflections are: i)   negative in aVR

ii)   usually positive in aVL

iii) usually positive in aVF.

In the precordial leads :

• Leads V_1, V_2 correspond roughly to the right atrium and ventricle.

• $V_4 - V_6$ correspond to the left ventricle.

• The P wave:

has maximum amplitude in V_1, diminishes, and is practically invisible in the left precordial leads.

• The Q wave:

is not present in $V_1 - V_3$,

is small or absent in $V_4 - V_6$.

• The R waves:

are small and S waves large in $V_1 - V_3$,

are large and the S waves small in $V_4 - V_6$.

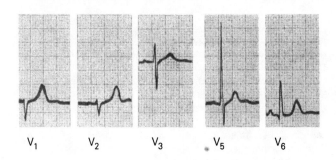

V_1 V_2 V_3 V_5 V_6

The P wave

The P wave is of low amplitude, less than 2.5 mm in lead II, of short duration (0.08-0.10 sec), electrical axis between 0° and 80°

The P wave shape varies between individuals:

Normal
• Upwards in I and II and downwards in aVR.

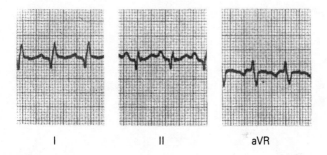

| I | II | aVR |

21

Abnormal

- In left atrial hypertrophy, abnormally long and bifid in II, biphasic with dominant downward component in V_1

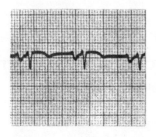
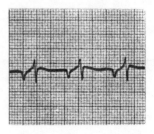

- In right atrial hypertrophy, abnormally tall in II for instance, cor pulmonale.

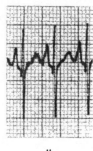
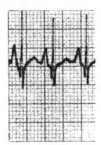

II   III

The P-R interval

Normal

• Duration 0.12 – 0.20 sec, varies inversely with heart rate.

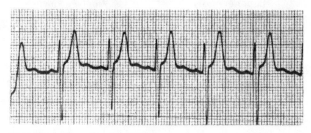

Shorter in sinus tachycardia

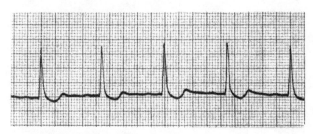

Longer in sinus bradycardia

Abnormal

- Short, in nodal rhythm (QRS normal).
- In Wolff–Parkinson–White syndrome (QRS abnormal).

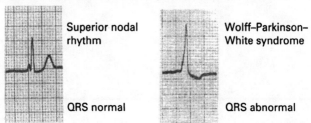

Superior nodal
rhythm

Wolff–Parkinson–
White syndrome

QRS normal

QRS abnormal

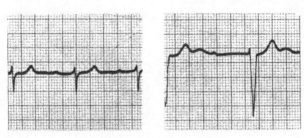

- Long, in 1st degree atrio-ventricular block.

The QRS complex

The QRS complex is of variable form, amplitude and sign, and of 0.06–0.10 sec duration.

Normal

- Upwards in I, II, V_5 and V_6
- Intermediate in the transition zone V_3 or V_1
- Downwards in aVR and V_1
- Up or down in aVL, aVF and III (depends on electrical axis).

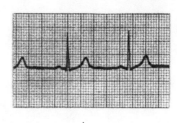

I

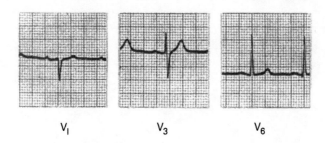

V_I V_3 V_6

QRS terminology

- First positive wave of a QRS is an R(r) wave
- Any second positive wave of a QRS is an R'(r') wave
- An initial negative wave is a Q(q) wave
- A negative following an R(r) wave is an S(s) wave
- A totally negative wave is a QS(qs) complex
- Relatively large waves are given **UPPER CASE** and relatively small waves **lower case** letters.

25

QRS dimensions

- At least one R wave in the precordial leads should equal or exceed 8 mm in height.
- The tallest R in the left precordial lead should not exceed 27 mm.
- The tallest R plus the deepest S in the precordial leads should not exceed 40 mm.
- Ventricular activation time should not exceed 0.03 sec.
- Total QRS duration should not exceed 0.10 sec.
- Any q waves present should not exceed 0.03 sec in duration and should have a depth greater than $1/4$ height of the ensuing R wave.

The QRS complex may, normally, take one of four forms in I or V_6, for example.

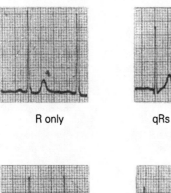

R only   qRs

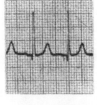   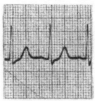

qR only   Rs only

The pathological QRS complex

Upwards

Abnormally large in I

in the Wolff–Parkinson–White syndrome, in complete left
bundle branch block and in left ventricular hypertrophy.

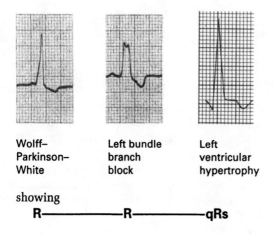

Wolff–   Left bundle   Left
Parkinson–   branch   ventricular
White   block   hypertrophy

showing

R—————R—————qRs

27

Downwards

- In myocardial infarct

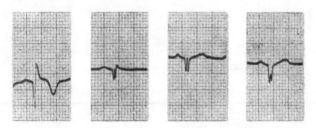

Dominantly negative waves (Q waves) in leads overlying a myocardial infarction

Intrinsic and intrinsicoid deflections

- The term intrinsic deflection was coined by Lewis to describe the abrupt, large deflection following the arrival of the stimulus at a myocardial electrode (direct recording).
- In clinical electrocardiography, the moment of activation of the myocardium near the exploring electrode at the peak of the R wave is the onset of what is known as the intrinsicoid deflection, as a result of which, its deflection returns to the baseline (ie the intrinsicoid deflection is the return (descending) part of the R wave). The intrinsicoid deflection time (also known as the ventricular activation time) is the time between the onset of the q wave and the peak of the R wave, in a left ventricular surface lead showing qR configuration.

  Normally, its value does not exceed 0.04 sec. It is prolonged in left ventricular hypertrophy.

The S–T interval

Normally isoelectric

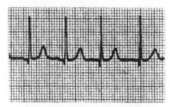

Abnormally depressed
• Prolonged depression in pericarditis
• Sagging in digitalis administration
• Potentially even more depressed in myocardial ischaemia.

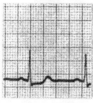 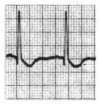 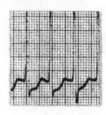

Pericarditis   Digitalis   Myocardial
ischaemia

Abnormally elevated

• In pericarditis

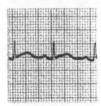

pericarditis

• More marked in the course of subpericardial lesions (commonly, ischaemia or infarction).

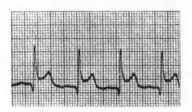 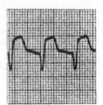

The T wave

Corresponds to repolarization of the ventricles.

Its maximum duration is 0.18 – 0.22 sec

Its shape is rather asymmetrical, the ascending segment is longer and shallower than the descending.

Normally upwards in I, V_6,

Normally downwards in aVR.

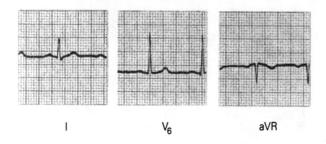

| I | V_6 | aVR |

Abnormally inverted

- In V_6 in left ventricular hypertrophy (1).
- In left bundle branch block over the left precordium (2) or right bundle branch block over the right precordium (3).
- In sub-epicardial ischaemia (4).

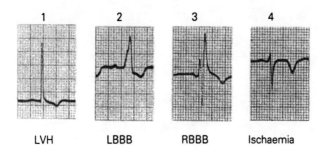

| LVH | LBBB | RBBB | Ischaemia |

The U wave

Upwards, follows T wave.
may or may not be visible, always small.

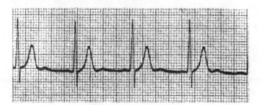

The electrical axis

The electrical axis of the heart, often simply referred to as "the axis", is usually held to refer to the mean frontal plane axis. Fundamentally, it relates to the predominant direction of depolarization of myocardium in the frontal plane. It is determined from inspection of the frontal plane leads (I, II, III, aVR, aVL and aVF) and has no connection with the precordial leads. In simple terms, it is closest to that frontal plane lead with the tallest upright QRS complex but this is not an adequate method of assessing the axis since the distribution of the limb leads within the frontal plane is not uniform. An understanding of the axis requires an initial understanding of the limb lead distribution in the frontal plane.

The figure shows the distribution of the limb leads in the frontal plane.

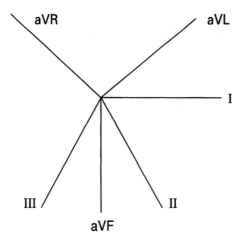

The electrical axis is determined with reference to a 360°
hexaxial system, with lead I arbitrarily assigned the value zero:

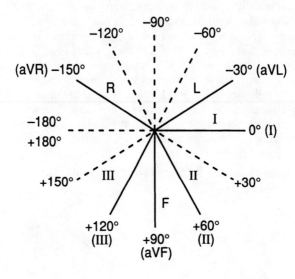

The normal frontal plane axis in the adult lies within the range −30° to +90° (travelling clockwise).

ECGs with axes beyond aVL (travelling counterclockwise) are said to show abnormal left axis deviation (LAD) and those with axes beyond aVF (travelling clockwise) are said to show abnormal right axis deviation (RAD) :

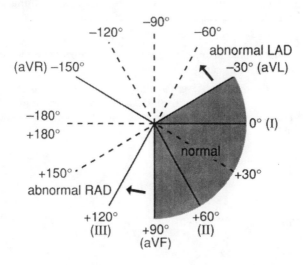

Axes in the region of +150° to − 120° cannot be classified on the basis of right or left axis deviation and this terminology is therefore of limited value.

The axis can be determined by simple inspection of the frontal plane lead as follows:

Example 1

i) First inspect the frontal plane leads and decide which lead has a QRS complex which is smallest and most equiphasic (eg lead aVL in figure).

   The axis is approximately at right angles to this lead.

ii) Determine the position of the lead in the hexaxial reference system (in this case –30°).

   The axis must lie at right angles to this, ie must be either –120° or +60°. These two positions are at opposite ends of the same straight line in the hexaxial reference system and are both at 90° to lead aVL.

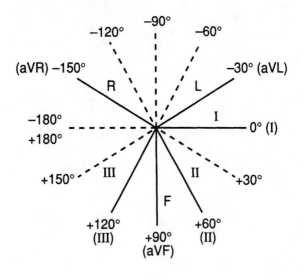

iii) One of the two positions lies on another lead – in this case, II. Inspect lead II of the ECG. The QRS must be large and will be either positive or negative. If it is positive (as here), the axis is towards lead II and is therefore +60° (as in this case). If lead II shows a deep negative QRS, the axis is away from lead II and would be –120°.

This technique gives the axis to the nearest 30°, which is adequate for most purposes.

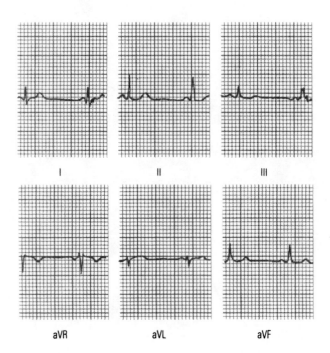

Example 2

i) The smallest, most equiphasic QRS is in aVR.

ii) The lead (aVR) is at −150°. The axis is, therefore, approximately at right angles to this (ie = +120°or −60°).

iii) One of these two positions (+120°) lies on another lead in this case, lead III. Inspection of lead III shows that QRS is predominantly negative in this lead. The left ventricle is, therefore, predominantly polarizing away from lead III and since we decided that it must depolarize either towards +120° or −60°, it must, in this case, be towards −60°.

The axis is therefore −60°, which is an abnormal degree of left axis deviation.

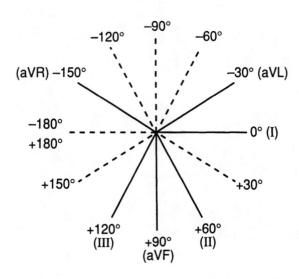

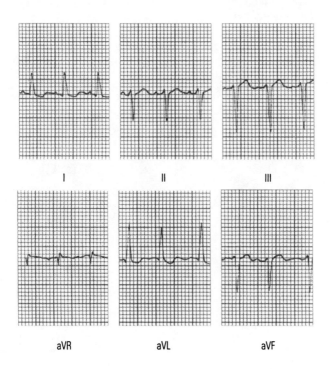

I

II

III

aVR

aVL

aVF

Example 3

i) Inspection of frontal plane leads reveals that aVR has the smallest (most equiphasic) QRS.

ii) The lead (aVR) is at –150°. The axis is, therefore, approximately at right angles to this (ie = +120° or –60°).

iii) One of these two positions (+120°) lies on another lead, in this case, lead III. Inspection of lead III shows that QRS is predominantly positive in this lead. The left ventricle is, therefore, predominantly polarizing towards lead III and since we decided that it must depolarize either towards +120° or –60°, it must, in this case, be towards +120°.

The axis is therefore +120°, which is an abnormal degree of right axis deviation.

If it were felt that lead I produced the most equiphasic QRS, then the calculated axis would be +90°, ie borderline right axis deviation.

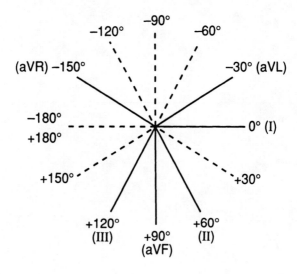

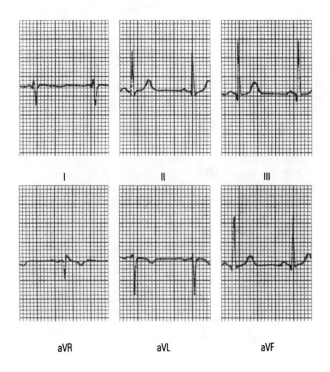

I II III

aVR aVL aVF

The significance of the axis

Hearts with a frontal plane QRS axis in the region of –30° to +30° are said to be horizontal hearts and those with axes in the region of +60° to +120° are said to be vertical hearts.

In infants, the normal axis lies in the range +90° to +150°. During childhood, the axis moves progressively to the left (becomes less positive) and in adult life it lies in the range –30° to +90° (travelling clockwise). In the 60s, the axis typically lies within the range 0° to –30° (travelling anticlockwise). When LBBB develops, the axis moves 15–30° to the left (so abnormal LAD will only develop if the axis was originally 0° to –30°) and in RBBB the axis moves 15–30° to the right (so abnormal right axis deviation will only develop if the axis was originally +60 to +90°).

The two commonest causes of abnormal LAD are inferior infarction and left anterior hemiblock (LAH). LAH implies block in the anterior division of the left bundle branch. LAH is, therefore, diagnosed by finding an axis more negative than –30°, in the absence of an abnormal q wave in aVF.

There are many causes of abnormal right axis deviation, including right ventricular hypertrophy, atrial septal defect (of the secundum type), pulmonary embolism and left posterior hemiblock (LPH). Because (unlike LAH) the other causes cannot be excluded on the ECG, the diagnosis of LPH cannot be made with certainty from the ECG.

Check Out Receipt

LAY, MICHAEL T.

tem: 33293003507763
itle: ABC of clinical electrocardiogra
hy
ue: 4/8/2013

tem: 33293003507920
itle: Electrocardiography pocket handb
ok
ue: 4/8/2013

otal Items: 2

The atrial hypertrophies

Left atrial hypertrophy

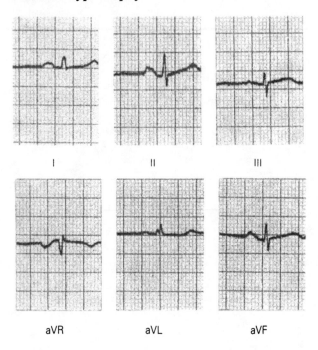

Shown typically in mitral stenosis but more commonly seen with left ventricular hypertrophy — giving bifid broad P waves in II and biphasic P waves, with dominant negative components in V_1.

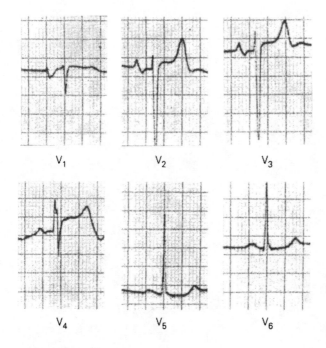

V_1 V_2 V_3

V_4 V_5 V_6

P waves broad and bifid in II
P waves have a dominant negative component in V_1. Both features
suggest left atrial hypertrophy.

Right atrial hypertrophy

Commonly seen in chronic cor pulmonale, altering the P waves to produce the P pulmonale.

Alterations of the P waves

• P is large and pointed in II–III.

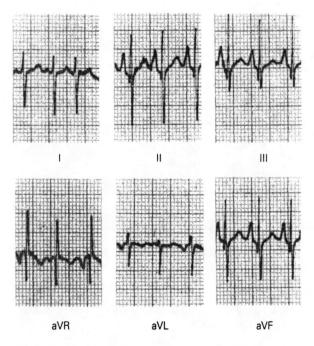

I   II   III

aVR   aVL   aVF

Tracing made on an infant aged one month with cyanotic congenital heart disease.

Right atrial hypertrophy, accompanied by a right ventricular hypertrophy

P wave
- Amplitude is increased ≥ 2.5 mm in II
- Tall and pointed in II, III and aVF.

QRS (indicates right ventricular hypertrophy)
- Abnormal right axis deviation
- Dominant R wave in V_1

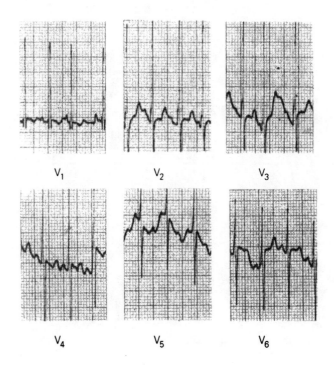

V_1 V_2 V_3

V_4 V_5 V_6

Bi-atrial hypertrophy

Uncommon, but seen with combined mitral and triscuspid stenosis, which causes hypertrophy of both atria, or with mitral stenosis and chronic pulmonary hypertension.

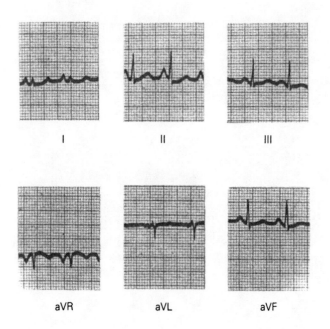

I

II

III

aVR

aVL

aVF

Modification of the P waves is a combination of the signs of left atrial hypertrophy and right atrial hypertrophy.

P wave
• Tall and pointed in I and II
• Large and bifid in III
• Biphasic in V_1 with dominant negative component.

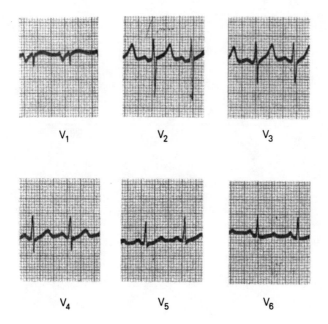

V_1 V_2 V_3

V_4 V_5 V_6

Left ventricular hypertrophy

Left ventricular hypertrophy occurs commonly in severe lesions of the aortic valves; aortic stenosis causes a concentric left ventricular hypertrophy with muscle hypertrophy and reduction of the volume of the chamber (systolic overload of the left ventricle).

Aortic incompetence shows a different appearance, called LVH diastolic overload, caused by a dilatation of the chamber, when the thickness of the wall is only slightly increased.

frontal plane   horizontal plane

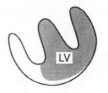 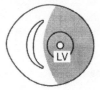

left ventricular hypertrophy
(systolic overload)

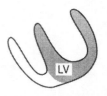

left ventricular hypertrophy
(diastolic overload)

- In the standard leads (I, II, III)

  Tall R waves in I (horizontal heart) or in II and III
  (vertical heart)

- In the unipolar limb leads
  tall R waves in aVL and I (horizontal heart) or in aVF
  (vertical heart).
- In the precordial leads
  rS complexes with deep S waves in V_1–V_3
  qR complexes with tall R waves in V_4–V_6,
  S-T depression and T inversion in V_5,V_6.

52

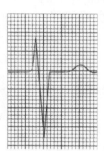

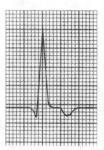

V_1–V_3
(irrespective of
heart position)
and in III and aVF
(horizontal heart)

V_4–V_6
(irrespective of
heart position)
and in I, aVL
(horizontal heart)
or in II, III, aVF
(vertical heart)

Left ventricular hypertrophy (systolic overload)

Limb leads

- QRS not necessarily abnormal but may have tall R in I, aVL (horizontal heart) or in II, III, aVF (vertical heart).
- S-T depression and asymmetrically negative T wave in I, II, III and aVF.

The changes are those of left ventricular hypertrophy. The voltage criteria for left ventricular are fulfilled in the precordial leads. The S-T, T changes in the limb leads and in the precordial leads are non-specific, but the probability is that they are secondary to the abnormal QRS complexes

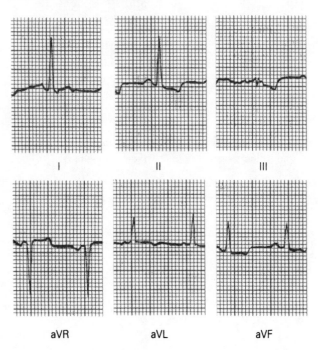

I   II   III

aVR   aVL   aVF

Precordial leads

Abnormally deep S waves in V_2 (R_{V_6} + S_{V_2} is greater than 40 mm). Non-specific S–T depression and T wave increases V_4-V_6. Delay in the onset of the intrinsic deflection in V_6.

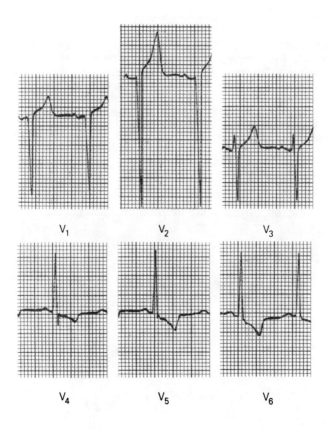

Left ventricular hypertrophy (diastolic overload)

Like the systolic overload pattern of LVH, this produces an increment of the R waves in V_6 and of the S waves in V_1 and V_2, with retardation of the intrinsicoid deflection in V_6, but there are minimal or no changes in the S–T segment or T waves (T waves remain upright in V_5 and V_6).

The precordial QRS complexes satisfy the voltage crtieria for left ventricular hypertrophy. In other respects, the record is within normal limits. The appearances are therefore consistent with diastolic overload of the left ventricle. It should be stated, however, that the distinction between systolic and diastolic overloads is ill-defined. It depends upon the (relative) prominence of S–T segment changes in addition to QRS voltage changes, which latter are common to both groups.

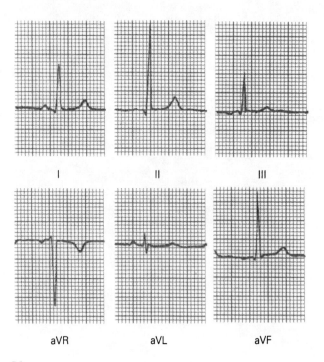

I	II	III

aVR	aVL	aVF

The criteria for LVH are :

(1) tallest precordial R > 27mm

(2) tallest precordial R plus deepest precordial S > 40mm

(3) ventricular activation time time > 0.03 sec (ie 0.04 sec or more)

(4) S-T depression and asymmetrical T wave inversion in V_5-V_6 and (when heart is horizontal) in I and aVL and (when heart is vertical) in II, F and III. The first three criteria are fulfilled in both systolic and diastolic overload patterns, the fourth criterion only in systolic overload.

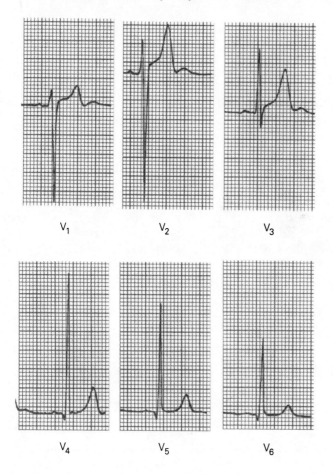

Right ventricular hypertrophy

Isolated right ventricular hypertrophy is typically found in patients with pulmonary hypertension or congenital pulmonary stenosis.

Limb leads

Right ventricular hypertrophy gives rise to:

- Abnormal right axis deviation.
- S-T depression and T wave inversion in those leads with a dominant R wave.

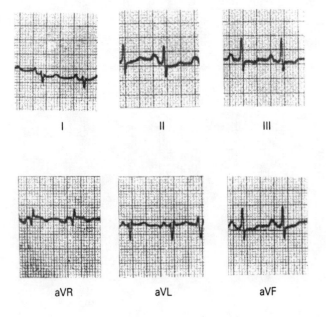

I   II   III

aVR   aVL   aVF

Precordial leads

- Dominant R wave in V_1 (ie R wave equals or exceeds S wave in this lead).
- Clockwise cardiac rotation.
- S-T depression and T wave inversion in V_1–V_3.

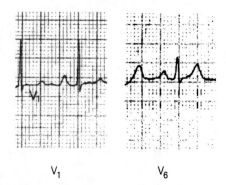

V_1 V_6

Right ventricular hypertrophy.
There is abnormal right axis deviation and a dominant R wave in V_1 and V_2. There is S-T depression and T wave inversion in V_1–V_3. Note the marked associated left atrial hypertrophy (dominantly negative P wave in V_1,V_2) —this patient had mitral stenosis

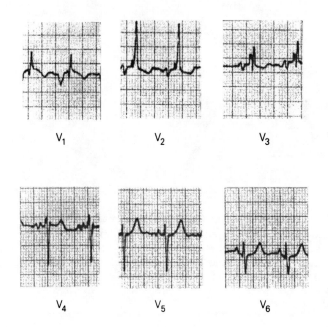

V_1 V_2 V_3

V_4 V_5 V_6

Biventricular hypertrophy

Biventricular hypertrophy is often a presumptive diagnosis since the electrical changes of LVH and RVH can cancel themselves out.

It may, however, be indicated by:
i) signs of LVH with **right** axis deviation
ii) signs of RVH with **left** axis deviation
iii) QRS evidence of both LVH and RVH in the precordial leads.

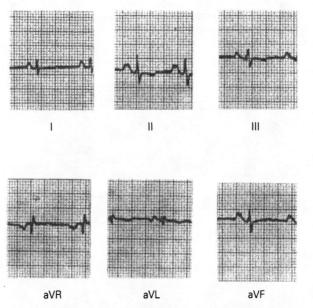

I   II   III

aVR   aVL   aVF

Mitral valve disease showing a hypertrophy of the four chambers of the heart. RAH in II and III ; LAH in I, II and V_1 and QRS changes of RVH seen in V_1, V_2, V_3 and of LVH in V_6, V_7. Here, it is valuable to take the outer precordial leads to help make the diagnosis. *[This is B.R.'s original diagnosis. It is rather bold in the confidence with which it recognises LVH and RAH —DJR.]*

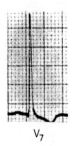

V_7

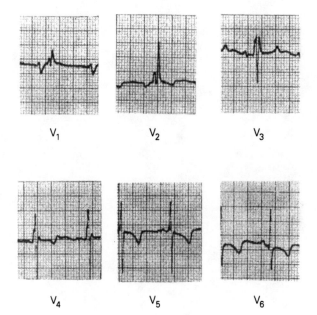

V_1 V_2 V_3

V_4 V_5 V_6

Electrical abnormalities in disease of the coronary circulation

Myocardial infarction

Myocardial infarction is caused by the occlusion of a coronary artery or one of its branches, leading to necrosis of the muscle territory normally supplied by the arterial branch.

The infarction can affect the three phases of the ventricular part of the ECG, that is to say,

- **QRS**

- **ST**

- **T**

Alteration of the QRS

- Infarction may be diagnosed when there is an abnormal Q wave, or QS complex.* an abnormal Q wave is one which is 0.04 sec or more in duration or which has a depth more than $\frac{1}{4}$ the height of the ensuing R wave.

- Occasionally, when a previous ECG is available for comparison, infarction may be demonstrated by significant loss of R wave height.

- In the absence of one or more of these **QRS changes** it is not possible to make a definitive diagnosis of myocardial infarction.

A QS complex is normal in a cavity lead (which aVR always is, which III is when the heart is horizontal, aVL is when the heart is vertical and V_1 is when there is clockwise rotation).

Necrosis of the myocardium = loss of wave height, abnormal qrs or QS complex

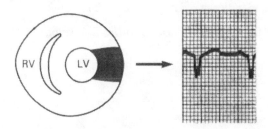

An electrical hole through the
the myocardium (QS complex)–
full-thickness infarct.

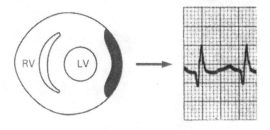

Necrosis
Major thickness sub-epicardial
necrosis (abnormal Q wave)

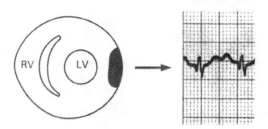

Minor thickness sub-epicardial
necrosis (loss of R wave height)

Alteration of the S–T

- This most frequently consists of an elevation of the segment which becomes convex upwards.
- This alteration indicates a zone of myocardial injury.

Myocardial injury = alterations in the S–T segment

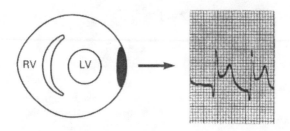

Anterior sub-epicardial lesion

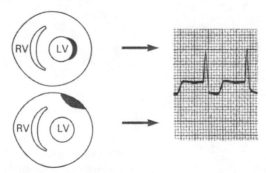

Anterior sub-endocardial lesion or a posterior, or an inferior, sub-epicardial lesion (reciprocal change)

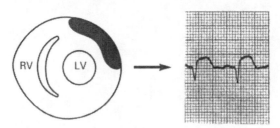

Posterior sub-epicardial lesion
(direct posterior lead – eg oesophageal lead)

- During the initial period of myocardial injury, the T wave is a part of the S–T segment, from which it cannot be distinguished.
- Later, it becomes distinct and negative, pointed and symmetrical.
- This indicates ischaemia.

Myocardial ischaemia = alterations in the T wave

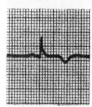

Ischaemic-type T wave changes
QRS suggests infarction

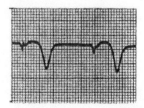

Ischaemic-type T wave changes
No evidence of infarction (V₆)

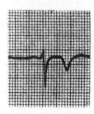

Ischaemic-type T wave changes
No evidence of infarction (necrosis) (V₂)

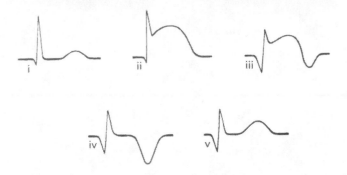

The figure above shows a diagrammatic representation of the evolution of the alterations of the complexes:

i)   Initial appearances before onset of infarction.

ii) Elevation of the S–T segment, concomitant with myocardial injury (hours after onset).

iii) Development of abnormal q waves and of T wave inversion (days after onset).

iv) Abnormal q wave present, S–T segment returns to normal, T wave inverted (weeks after onset).

v)   Abnormal Q wave present, S–T and T waves have returned to normal (months after onset).

• The most frequent definitive sign of necrosis is the Q wave.

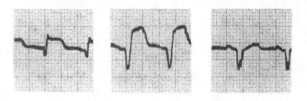

From the various leads in which the abnormalities of the ventricular complexes are shown, one can deduce the appropriate location of the infarct.

Systematically, one distinguishes three principal types of infarcts.

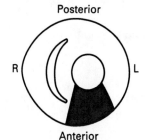

• Antero-septal infarct
This damages the anterior wall of the left ventricle reaching more or less to the interventricular septum.
The electrical alterations appear in :

V_2, V_3, V_4 and sometimes V_1.

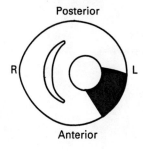

• Antero-lateral infarct
This damages the anterior wall of the left ventricle to its internal surface and extends along the left border of the heart as far as the apex.
The electrical alterations are seen in

V_5, V_6, I and aVL.

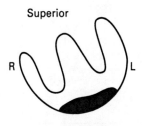

• The inferior infarct
This damages the posterior diaphragmatic wall of the left ventricle.
The electrical alterations are seen in
II, III, aVF sometimes V_6.

69

Extensive anterior myocardial infarction

The appearance of scarring in an extensive anterior myocardial infarction.

- QS complex in V_2, V_3, V_4
- Abnormal, small r waves in V_2.
- Abnormal Q waves in V_5 and V_6.

There are also abnormal q waves in II and aVF, indicating inferior infarction.

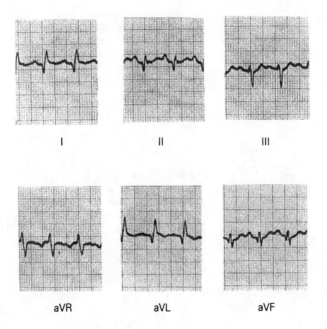

I   II   III

aVR   aVL   aVF

Less proximal left coronary block

RC = *Right coronary*
LC = *Left coronary*
Circ = *Circumflex*
PD = *Posterior descending*
AD = *Anterior descending*
D1,D2 = *Diagonal*

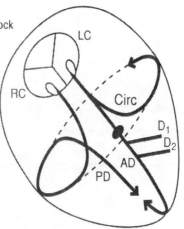

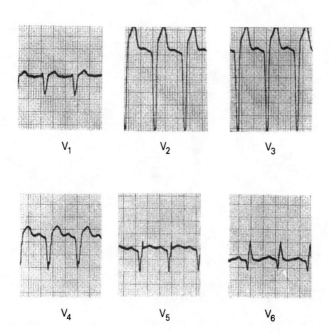

V₁ V₂ V₃

V₄ V₅ V₆

Antero-septal myocardial infarction

Antero-septal myocardial necrosis, the QS wave of transmural necrosis from V_1-V_4.

Extensive anterior ischaemia from V_2 to V_6 and in I and aVL.

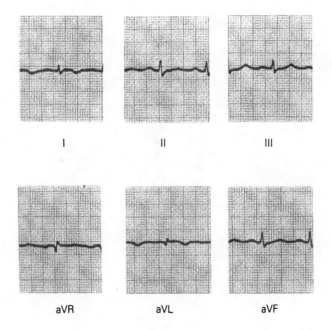

I II III

aVR aVL aVF

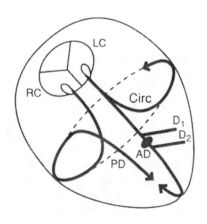

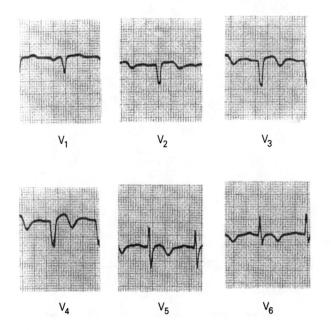

Antero-lateral myocardial infarction

Abnormal Q waves in I, aVL and V_6 and abnormally low R wave voltage in V_3 and V_4 from the lateral sub-endocardial necrosis.

- QS complexes in V_5 from the apical transmural necrosis.
- Non-specific S-T,T changes in I, II, aVL and V_3–V_6, probably indicative of sub-epicardial ischaemia.

(The R waves are of low voltage in V_1–V_3. This is not necessarily abnormal, but if the R waves in these leads were formerly taller it would indicate more extensive infarction and a more proximal site for the lesion).

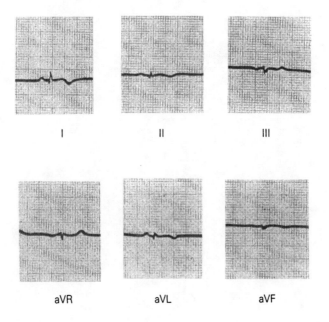

I   II   III

aVR   aVL   aVF

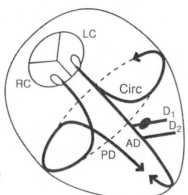

RC = Right coronary
LC = Left coronary
Circ = Circumflex
PD = Posterior descending
AD = Anterior descending
D1,D2 = Diagonal

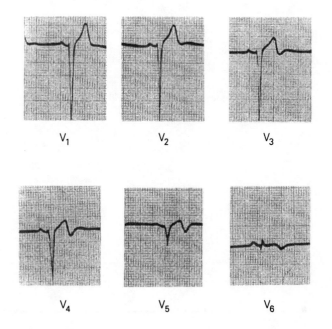

Inferior myocardial infarction

Inferior myocardial infarction with pathological Q waves in II, III and aVF.

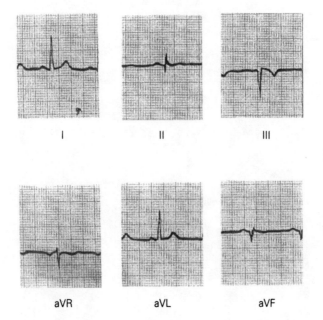

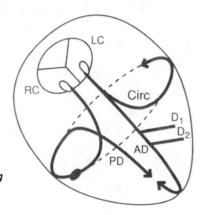

RC = Right coronary
LC = Left coronary
Circ = Circumflex
PD = Posterior descending
AD = Anterior descending
D1,D2 = Diagonal

No abnormality in the precordial leads

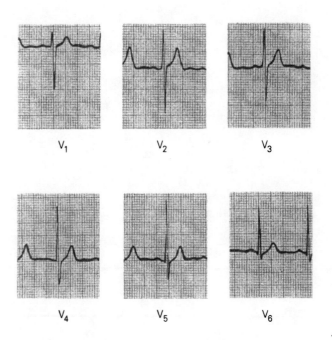

An electrocardiographic recording taken during an acute attack of angina may show:

- No acute change.

- (Commonly) S–T depression (as here) indicative of sub-endocardial ischaemia in the corresponding area of myocardium (in this case S–T depression in V_3-V_6, I and aVL indicates antero-lateral sub-endocardial ischaemia).

- (Occasionally) deep, symmetrical T wave inversion indicative of sub-epicardial ischaemia in the corresponding area of myocardium.

- (Very rarely) S–T elevation (Prinzmetal's variant) which usually indicates the presence of a tight stenosis situated proximally in a coronary artery (often the left anterior descending artery) and often associated with spasm in the vessel.

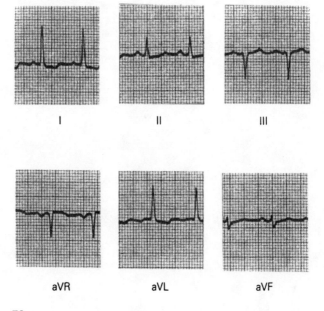

I   II   III

aVR   aVL   aVF

Antero-lateral sub-endocardial ischaemic lesion

- Anterior sub-endocardial ischaemic lesion with sagging of the S–T in V_3 to V_6 and the T wave pointed and positive in V_2 to V_6.

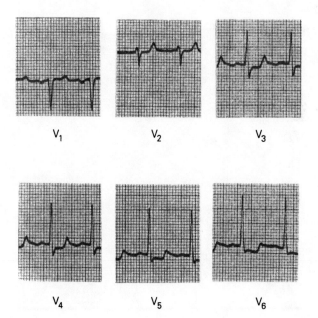

V_1 V_2 V_3

V_4 V_5 V_6

Between anginal attacks the electrocardiogram may show evidence of continuing myocardial ischaemia (as described on page 78) but often shows no evidence of acute ischaemia, in which case it is often normal, or shows evidence only of previous myocardial infarction.

Extensive sub-epicardial anterior myocardial ischaemia

Electrocardiographic tracing taken in the absence of acute angina, showing an extensive anterior, sub-epicardial ischaemia (T wave negative and pointed in all the leads exploring the left ventricle).

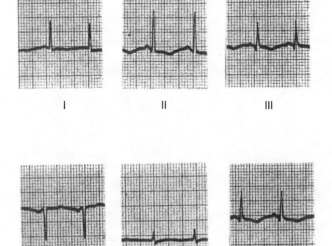

I   II   III

aVR   aVL   aVF

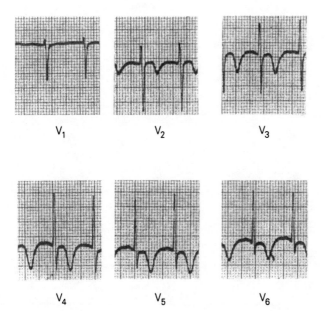

V_1 V_2 V_3

V_4 V_5 V_6

81

Electrical disturbances in the disorders of conduction and activation

It is appropriate to begin this section with a reminder of the pathway of the spread of the depolarization process within the heart.

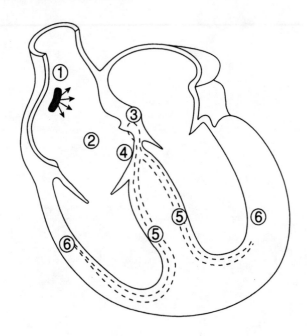

The pathway of depolarization in the cardiac muscle

- The stimulus which will initiate the contraction of the heart begins in a node of tissue called the sino-atrial node (1), situated in the right atrium at the junction of the atrium and the superior vena cava.

- In the atria there is no continuous pathway of specialized conduction cells but there appear to be some general preferential pathways of conduction via the atrial myocardium (2).

- On arrival at the atrio-ventricular junction, the excitation wave passes through the atrio-ventricular node (3) which, like the sino-atrial node, has intrinsic rhythmicity but which also has the important property of slow conduction, which, in normal circumstances optimizes the time between atrial and ventricular activation (and therefore contraction).

- From here, the stimulus goes by a unique route, the only bridge between the atria and the ventricles; the bundle of His (4).

- At the top of the interventricular septum, this bundle divides into two branches, right and left (5), which carry the excitation to the corresponding ventricles (6).

Normal and abnormal rhythm initiated at the SA node

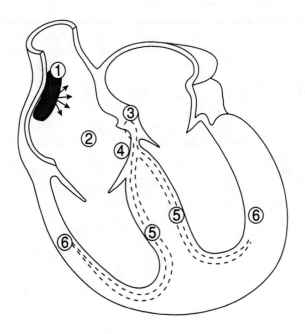

84

Sinus tachycardia and bradycardia

Sinus tachycardia

Sinus tachycardia means sinus rhythm with a rate of more than 100 beats/min. The rate can vary within large limits between 100-180 beats/min (or even beyond this, during peak physical exercise). The PR and QT intervals shorten according to the speed of the tachycardia but remain within physiological limits. The T waves are reduced in amplitude; S–T segment undergoes a downward sag (actually due to a prominent atrial repolarization wave (Ta wave), which begins before the QRS complex). Tachycardia is physiological in the child until the age of six. In the adult, sympathatonia, physical exercise, emotion, digestion, fever, shock, anaemia, or hyperthyroidism may cause tachycardia.

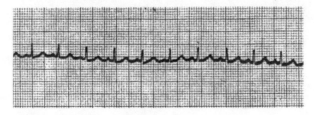

Sinus tachycardia at 130 beats/min

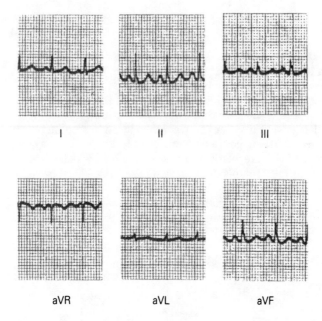

I II III

aVR aVL aVF

Sinus tachycardia at 130 beats/min.

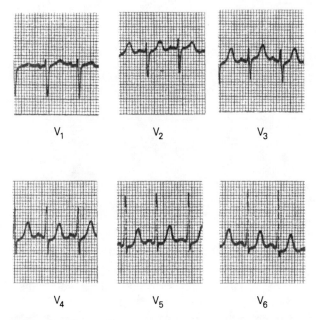

V₁   V₂   V₃

V₄   V₅   V₆

Sinus bradycardia

Sinus bradycardia means sinus rhythm with a rate less than
60 beats/min. The rate can vary between 35 and 60, but it is
rarely less than 45 beats/min; being the opposite of a
tachycardia, the PR and QT intervals lengthen. Found in
athletes and in vagotonia.

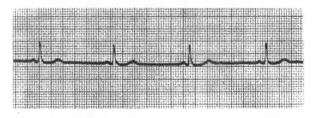

Sinus bradycardia at 48 beats/min.

Sinus arrhythmias, sinus arrest, sino-atrial block and AV nodal escape

Sinus arrhythmia

Sinus arrhythmia means sinus rhythm with varying rates. This non-pathogenic rhythm is characterized by alternate acceleration and slowing of the heart rate by respiration and is most often produced in the infant, young adult and in the elderly.

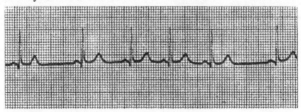

Physiological respiratory sinus arrhythmia

Sinus arrest

Sinus arrest means transient cessation of SA nodal activity. This gives rise to a transient pause between sinus beats. If the pause is prolonged, there will usually be an AV nodal (junctional) escape beat. Typically, however, the pause is less than twice the normal (ie preceding) sinus interval.

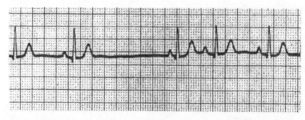

Sinus arrhythmia with a pause (probably due to sinus arrest, since the pause is not an integral multiple of the preceding sinus interval but difficult to be sure because of the underlying irregularity of the sinus rhythm)

Sino-atrial block

Sino-atrial block implies normal sinus node depolarization with failure of transmission of the depolarization to the atrial myocardium. If the SA block occurs in relation to a single beat, the resulting pause is exactly twice the normal (preceding) sinus beat interval.

The ECG appearances of sinus arrest and sino-atrial block are similar but not identical. In sino-atrial block, the pause is an integral (whole number) multiple of the preceding sino-atrial depolarization interval. In sinus arrest, the interval is not an integral multiple unless the period of arrest happens to be precisely the same as the sinus interval. If the basic sinus interval is irregular, the distinction cannot be made.

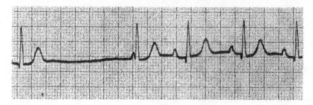

Sinus arrest or sino-atrial block (cannot be distinguished since regularity or otherwise of sinus rhythm prior to the pause cannot be seen) with AV nodal escape. There is AV nodal escape with a nodally initiated QRS occurring before the half-formed P wave can transmit through the AV node

AV nodal escape

AV nodal escape usually occurs when there is a delay in the arrival of the sinus-initiated beat at the AV node. This commonly occurs in sinus arrest, occasionally in sino-atrial block and rarely during pauses in sinus arrhythmia.

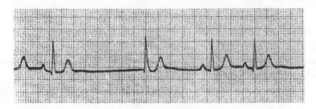

Example of AV nodal escape following sinus arrest

Sinus extrasystole

Non-pathogenic sinus extrasystole

The stimulus arises prematurely in the sino-atrial node and leads to a slightly early ventricular contraction, not deformed, preceded by a normal P wave, with normal PR interval.

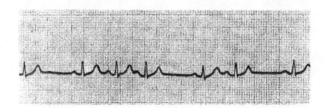

Frequent sinus extrasystoles

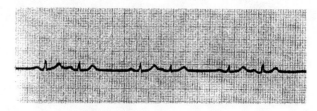

Coupled sinus extrasystoles

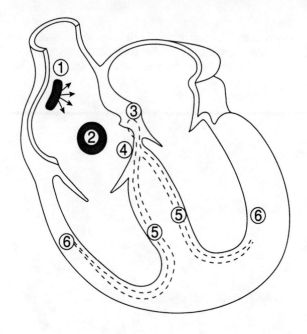

Atrial tachycardia

In atrial tachycardia there is a rapid, regular atrial rate (usually at 160–250 beats/min).When the atrial rate is less than 180 beats/min there is usually 1:1 atrio-ventricular conduction. At faster rates there is usually 2:1 atrio-ventricular conduction. If there is atrio-ventricular node dysfunction or if drugs blocking the AV node are used (eg digitalis, beta-blockers, verapamil or diltiazem) there may be 3:1 or 4:1 atrio-ventricular block. Atrial tachycardia is also discussed under 'paroxysmal supraventricular tachycardia', page 98.

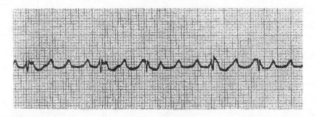

Atrial tachycardia (AT). Regular P waves are seen at 210 beats/min. There is an iso-electric interval between consecutive P waves. The slower rate and consequent iso-electric interval distinguish the rhythm from atrial flutter where the rate is 280–300 beats/min. The QRS rate is substantially slower, there being alternating 4:1 and 3:1 atrio-ventricular block

Atrial flutter and fibrillation

Atrial flutter and fibrillation are two disorders of rhythm characterized by an atrial tachycardia, in which the activation of the atria is ectopic and proceeds at a rate which is very much higher than normal:

Between 200–400 beats/min and regular for flutter

and between 400–700 beats/min and irregular for fibrillation.

- In flutter, the time interval between consecutive flutter waves is shorter than the AV nodal refractory period (recovery time) and therefore (typically) every alternate atrial depolarization is conducted to the ventricles. The atrial rate is 300 (and regular) and the ventricular rate is 150 (and regular), ie there is 2:1 atrio-ventricular conduction block. With the use of drugs which interfere with AV nodal conduction (eg digoxin, beta-blockers, verapamil and diltiazem) or with vagal activity, the degree of AV block may increase to 3:1 (with a ventricular rate of 100 beats/min) or to 4:1 (with a ventricular rate of 75 beats/min) or to even greater degrees of block.

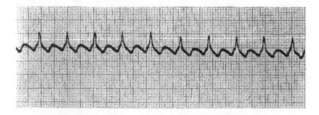

2:1 flutter with an atrial rate of 280 and a ventricular rate of 140 beats/min

- In atrial fibrillation, the atrial stimuli are very numerous (400–700 beats/min) and this results in grossly disorganized activity of the atrial myocardium, which shows itself by fibrillation waves, clearly seen in V_1 (page 96).

The ventricles respond irregularly to these multiple disorganized atrial stimuli: the atrio-ventricular node is blocked to a proportion of them. This results in an irregular ventricular rate. Generally, the ventricular rate is rapid, producing a complete tachyarrhythmia.

Atrial fibrillation

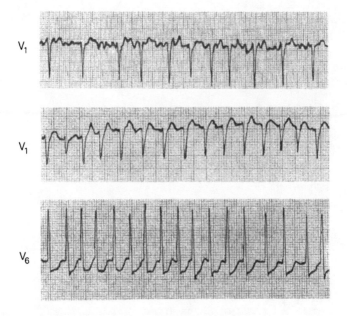

Atrial fibrillation with a rapid ventricular rate.

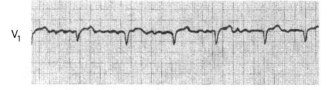

Atrial fibrillation with a slow ventricular rate

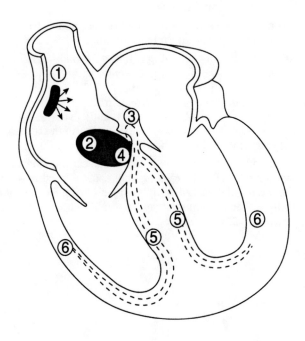

Paroxysmal supraventricular tachycardia

This is a broad term encompassing several varieties of episodic tachycardias, arising at sites superior to the bifurcation of the His bundle. Most are due to re-entrant circuits in closed loops of excitable myocardium. There is a variety of possible sites and mechanisms for the re-entrant loops, which sustain the arrhythmias, but the three commonest electrocardiographic categories of tachycardias involve:

i) Re-entrant circuits entirely within the AV node (atrio-ventricular nodal re-entrant tachycardia, AVNRT),

ii) Re-entrant circuits involving both the AV node and an accessory atrio-ventricular conduction pathway (atrio-ventricular re-entrant tachycardia, AVRT) (see under Wolff–Parkinson–White syndrome, p128). These re-entrant circuits involve small areas of atrial and of ventricular myocardium lying between the AV node and the accessory pathway at the proximal and distal ends,

iii) Re-entrant circuits within the atrial myocardium (atrial tachycardia, AT). The relative frequences of occurrence of these three electrocardiographic types of supraventricular tachycardias are (approximately) AVNRT 50%; AVRT 35%; AT 15%.

In general, it is possible to distinguish between these three common varieties of supraventricular tachycardias **but it is not always possible to make these distinctions.**

The main principles of the electrocardiographic diagnosis are as follows:

i)   Tachycardias associated with narrow (≯0.10sec) QRS complexes are supraventricular.

ii) Supraventricular tachycardias will have narrow QRS complexes unless (a) there is pre-existing bundle branch block or intraventricular conduction defect, (b) there is ventricular pre-excitation during the tachycardia, (c) there is functional (tachycardia-related) bundle branch block.

iii) In cases of **AVNRT**, depolarization spreads from the re-entrant circuit within the AV node to the atria and to the ventricles virtually simultaneously and the P waves (which are actually negative since depolarizations spread retrogradely through the atria) are hidden in the QRS complex. The ECG appearances are therefore those of rapid, regular, narrow QRS complexes with no P wave visible.

iv) In cases of **AVRT**, conduction within the re-entrant circuit is usually from atria to ventricles via the AV node (orthodromic conduction), then from the distal AV node to the distal part of the atrio-ventricular accessory pathway via the small intervening segment of ventricular myocardium, then retrogradely via the accessory pathway, then from the proximal end of the accessory pathway to the proximal part of the AV node via the small intervening segment of atrial myocardium. Atrial myocardial depolarization is therefore initiated after ventricular myocardial depolarization and is retrograde. The P waves are therefore negative in lead II and are seen first after the QRS (or in the terminal part of the QRS). The ECG appearances of AVRT are usually therefore those of rapid, regular, narrow QRS complexes with small negative deflections (P waves) visible at the end of, or just after, the QRS complexes. Since both atrial and ventricular myocardium are involved in the re-entrant circuit, there is always a 1:1 atrio-ventricular ratio (ie, there is one QRS to each P wave).

v) In cases of **AT**, the re-entrant circuit lies somewhere in the atrial myocardium and gives rise to P waves, the shape and size of which depend on the location and size of the re-entrant loop. Rapid but regular (often recognizably abnormal) P waves occur, and if the P wave rate exceeds 150 beats/min (as it usually does), the time interval between consecutive P waves will be less than the AV nodal refractory period (recovery time) and intermittent failure of atrio-ventricular conduction will result. Most typically, there is 2:1 AV conduction failure, giving a ventricular rate of half the atrial rate (though in the presence of vagal activity or of drugs like digoxin, beta-blockers, verapamil or diltiazem, greater degrees of AV block may occur). The ECG appearances, therefore, are typically of rapid, regular, narrow QRS complexes with regular, upright, abnormal P waves. It is important to note that alternate P waves are often partly obscured by QRS complexes. In tachycardias with a rate of 150 beats/min and narrow QRS complexes, the chances are high that the rhythm is atrial flutter or tachycardia with 2:1 AV block. Atrial flutter is best regarded as a special case of atrial tachycardia in which the atrial rate is 300 beats/min and the ventricular rate is typically 150 beats/min. Atrial tachycardia has a slower atrial rate than atrial flutter. Typically, the atrial rate is 180–240 beats/min again, usually with 2:1 atrio-ventricular block. The slower atrial rate results in a brief iso-electric (horizontal) interval between consecutive P waves (except where this interval is interrupted by QRS complexes) which differs from the situation in atrial flutter where each flutter wave immediately follows its predecessor without an iso-electric interval.

AVNRT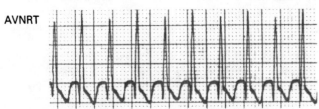

Chest monitoring lead. Paroxysmal (re-entrant) junctional tachycardia of the intra-AV nodal type, ie AVNRT. Ventricular rate 205 beats/min and regular. No P waves identified. QRS complexes are not abnormally wide T waves are inverted

100

AVRT

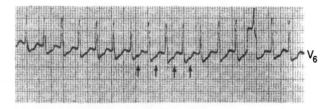

Narrow QRS tachycardia, regular at 210 beats/min. Small P waves
are seen just after each QRS

AVRT

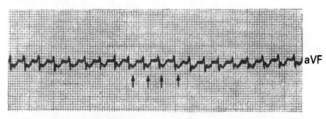

Narrow QRS tachycardia, regular at 250 beats/min. Small P waves
are seen just after each QRS (arrows)

Atrial tachycardia

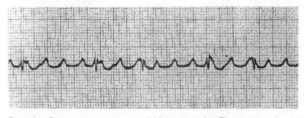

Regular P waves are seen at 210 beats/min. There is an iso-electric
interval between consecutive P waves. The slower rate and
consequent iso-electric interval distinguish the rhythm from atrial
flutter where the rate is 280–300 beats/min. The QRS rate is
substantially slower, there being alternating 4:1 and 3:1 atrio-
ventricular block

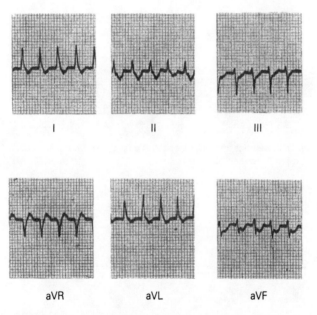

I II III

aVR aVL aVF

Atrio-ventricular re-entrant tachycardia (AVRT). The QRS complexes are narrow and there is a regular tachycardia at 214 beats/min. Inverted P waves are seen after the QRS (best seen in I, II, aVF and V_6). The appearances are typical of AVRT.

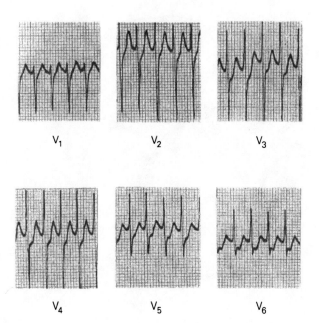

V_1 V_2 V_3

V_4 V_5 V_6

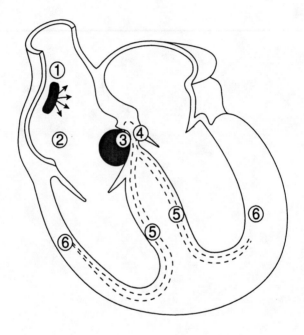

When the sino-atrial node does not give rise to a spontaneous depolarization within the (usually longer) time taken by the atrio-ventricular node to give rise to its spontaneous depolarization, the atrio-ventricular node usually takes command, giving rise to a **nodal rhythm.** This is an escape rhythm since the AV node (which has intrinsic rhythmicity like the SA node) is normally prematurely depolarized by the incident depolarization arriving from the sino-atrial node.

Depolarization spreads from the AV node, antegradely to the ventricles (giving a normal QRS complex) and retrogradely to the atria (giving an inverted P wave). The retrograde atrial depolarization may occur prior to, during or after the QRS (depending on relative conduction times) and the relationship may vary on a beat-by-beat basis. Sometimes, there is no conduction to the atria and no P waves occur.

Nodal rhythm occurs when the sino-atrial node is inhibited, for example, during vagal hyperactivity (in pain or emotion-sensitive individuals and in athletes), in the sick sinus syndrome (intrinsic depression of SA activity) and in response to some anti-arrhythmic drugs.

It may also occur in infective myocarditis (acute polyarthritic rheumatism, typhoid, diphtheria) or in myocardial infarction.

Nodal rhythm

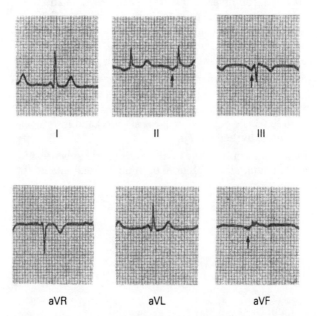

I   II   III

aVR   aVL   aVF

Negative P waves are clearly visible in II and can be seen in III, aVF and V_2–V_4 (arrows). The P waves seen before the QRS complex indicate that in this case (at least at the time of the recording) spread of depolarization from the AV node reaches the atria before the ventricles. The rate is usually slower than this in nodal rhythm. This suggests that, in this case, the AV nodal depolarization rate has been accelerated (rather than the more usual explanation that the sino-atrial rate falls – when the nodal rhythm is an escape rhythm)

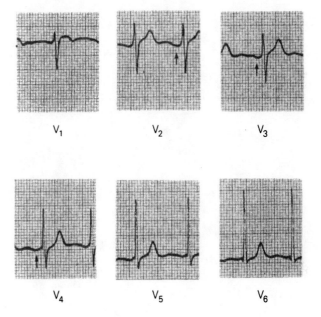

V_1 V_2 V_3

V_4 V_5 V_6

Nodal rhythm

The rate is slow. It is difficult to be sure whether or not P waves are visible but it is possible that the slight deflection seen towards the end of the QRS complexes (arrows) represents regular P waves

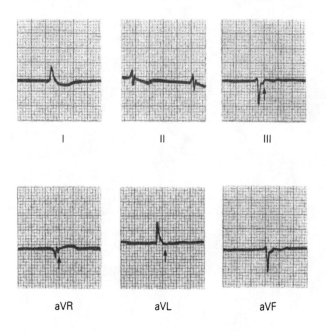

I

II

III

aVR

aVL

aVF

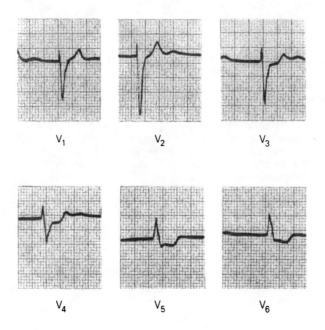

V_1

V_2

V_3

V_4

V_5

V_6

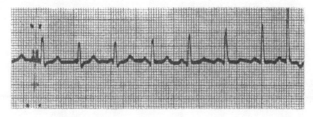

V_2

Nodal rhythm giving way to sinus rhythm

The first three beats are nodal rhythm, P waves then return
(presumably the sino-atrial nodal depolarization frequency has
increased) and the sinus rhythm returns. The last QRS is a
ventricular premature beat. The fourth beat is probably of nodal
rather than sinus origin since the P–R interval is short, suggesting
that spontaneous depolarization of the AV node occurred before
the sinus depolarization (indicated by the upright P wave) could
reach and suppress the AV node

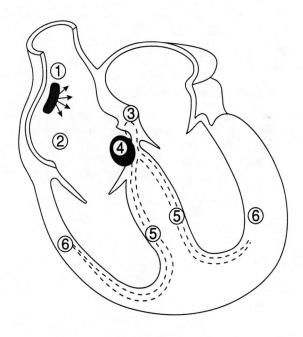

The atrio-ventricular block (heart block)

Atrio-ventricular block results from a partial or complete
failure of conduction through those parts of the conducting
tissue which normally provide the only electrical pathway
between atrial myocardium and ventricular myocardium (the
AV node and the His bundle).

There are three degrees (grades) of heart block:

• First degree heart block.

• Second degree heart block.

• Third degree (complete) heart block.

First degree incomplete heart block

The conduction in the AV node is abnormally slow but not
interrupted. The ECG shows a constant, prolonged (>0.20 sec)
P–R interval. The P–R interval is measured from the beginning
of the P wave to the beginning of the QRS complex.

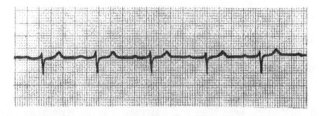

First degree heart block. P–R = 0.26 sec and constant

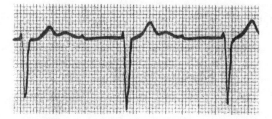

First degree heart block. P–R = 0.56 sec and constant

113

Second degree atrio-ventricular block

Whereas in first degree heart block each sinus beat is successfully conducted to the ventricles (albeit after an abnormally long interval), and in third degree heart block no sinus beats are conducted to the ventricles, the characteristic of second degree heart block is that some sinus beats are conducted to the ventricles and some are not. There are two types of second degree block and one special situation, (in which it is not possible to tell which type is present).

Type I second degree atrio-ventricular block is also known as **the Wenckebach phenomenon** or as **Möbitz type I block.** In this rhythm, there is progressive atrio-ventricular conduction **delay** until **failure** of conduction occurs for one beat, following which conduction is transiently normalized, only for progressive conduction failure to recur. Typically, the P-R interval shows a progressive increase until the P wave is not followed by a QRS complex. The cycle then repeats itself. In any one such cycle there is one more P wave than the number of QRS complexes. The ratios could be 3:2, 4:3, 5:4, etc (though these three are the commonest) and the ratios may vary spontaneously, eg 3:2, 3:2, 3:2, 4:3, 3:2, etc.

Type I block is usually innocent and transient. It is often related to vagal hyperactivity and can be seen in the resting ECG of athletes.

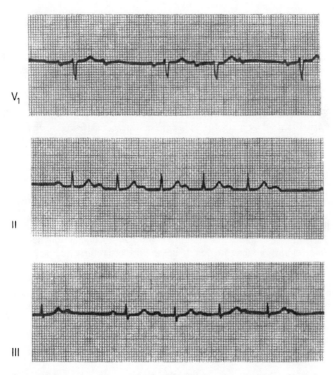

V₁

II

III

Second degree atrio-ventricular block, showing the Wenckebach
phenomenon, characterized by a steady lengthening of the P–R
interval until the P wave occurs without a ventricular response

Type II second degree atrio-ventricular block (also known as **Möbitz type II second degree AV block**) differs from type I block in that the P–R interval is **constant** (whether normal or prolonged) in the beats prior to the transient conduction failure.

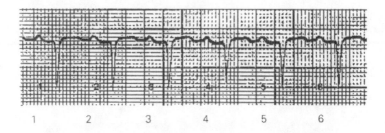

Sinus rhythm with first degree heart block and type II second degree atrio-ventricular block. The first three beats show sinus rhythm with a slightly prolonged but constant P-R interval. The fourth P wave is not followed by a QRS complex (failure of atrio-ventricular conduction). After the transient conduction failure the rhythm returns to first degree heart block

Type II second degree block is not innocent and rarely occurs in normal subjects. Its presence carries with it a significant risk of the development of complete heart block.

The special case of 2:1 AV block deserves consideration. In this situation, alternate P waves are conducted to the ventricles and alternate ones are not. The ECG provides no means of knowing whether there was type I (usually a conduction problem in the AV node) or type II (a conduction problem inferior to the AV node) block. More commonly, however, it is type II (demonstrable only by electrophysiological study).

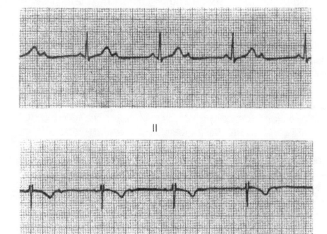

II

V_1

2:1 atrio-ventricular block. Only alternate P waves are followed by QRS complexes

Third degree atrio-ventricular block (complete heart block)

In third degree or complete atrio-ventricular block, there is total failure of conduction from atria to ventricles. The atrial and ventricular rates are therefore completely independent (ie there is atrio-ventricular dissociation). The atrial rhythm is most commonly sinus (but could be atrial flutter, atrial fibrillation, atrial tachycardia or, indeed, any atrial rhythm). When the atrial rhythm is of sinus origin, the atrial rate is increased as a result of reflex baroreceptor activation consequent on the slow ventricular rate. The ventricular rate is slow and the ventricular rhythm is an escape rhythm with a rate in the region of 20–70 beats/min. The QRS rate is usually regular (at the escape rate). The shape and width of the QRS complexes (and the escape rate) are related to the location of the ventricular escape pacemaker, ie of the ventricular cell with the fastest intrinsic rate. When this cell is situated close to the AV node, the QRS complexes are narrow and the rate is 50–70 beats/min. When the escape rhythm arises from distal Purkinje cells, the QRS is wide and the rate is 20–40 beats/min.

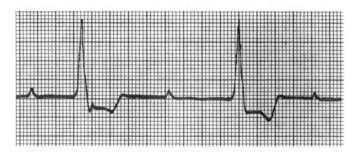

The QRS rate is regular and slow and the QRS complexes are abnormally wide. The P wave rate is regular and greater than the QRS rate. There is complete atrio-ventricular dissociation (ie P waves and QRS complexes are independent). The second P wave is seen just after the first QRS and the fourth P wave is hidden in the second QRS. The rhythm is sinus with complete heart block (as is usual in this condition, the ventricular rhythm is an escape rhythm)

At the level of the branches of the bundle of His,
ie Bundle Branch Block

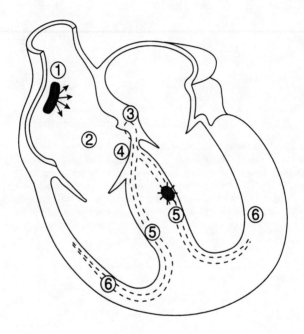

Complete bundle branch blocks

Complete left bundle branch block

Left bundle branch block fundamentally alters the shape and dimensions of the QRS complexes in all leads and does so to such an extent that, in the presence of left bundle branch block, it is no longer possible to recognize myocardial infarction or ventricular hypertrophy from inspection of the QRS complexes. It is unwise to attempt a further diagnosis from the electrocardiogram (except to comment on the P wave, the cardiac rhythm and the frontal plane QRS axis) since there are also inevitable major secondary changes in the S-T segment and T waves. The reason for the dramatic changes induced by left bundle branch block is that this condition results in (a) reversal of the direction of each QRS complex and (b) delay in depolarization of the left ventricle. The initial direction of the QRS complex and the timing and direction of left ventricular depolarization are the two most important determinants of the normal ECG.

The three criteria needed for a diagnosis of left bundle branch block (LBBB), all of which must be fulfilled, are:

- i) A total QRS duration of 0.12 sec (3 small squares) or more.
- ii) Absence of an initial q wave in the leads facing the left ventricle (V_4–V_6, I, aVL).
- iii) Absence of an rsR' in V_1 (the presence of which would point to right bundle branch block (RBBB)).

There are usually pronounced S-T segments and T wave changes, secondary to the QRS abnormality, giving S–T depression and negative T waves in those leads where the QRS is upright and elevated S–T segments and tall T waves in those leads where the QRS is negative.

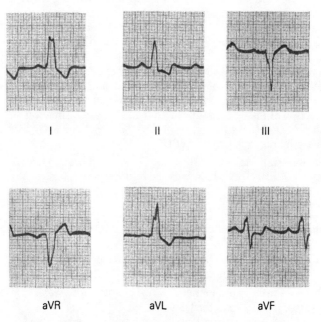

I II III

aVR aVL aVF

Complete block of the left branch of the bundle of His:

- Increase of the QRS to 0.12 sec (seen in I, aVR, aVL, V_2–V_6)
- No initial q wave in I, aVL, V_4–V_6
- No rsR′ in V_1

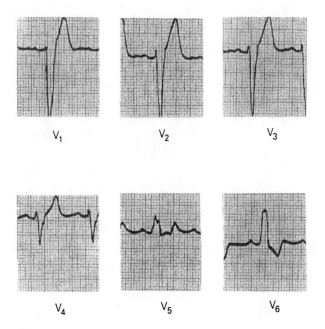

V_1 V_2 V_3

V_4 V_5 V_6

Complete right bundle branch block

In right bundle branch block, the changes to the QRS complexes (and therefore the secondary changes to the S–T segments and T waves) are much less dramatic than in LBBB. The initial direction of the QRS complexes and the timing of left ventricular depolarization are unaltered. The fundamental change is a delay in depolarization of the right ventricle. This results in a change in the QRS, in V_1, from an rS complex to an rSr' complex and in V_6, from a qR complex to a qRs complex.

The criteria for the diagnosis of RBBB (both of which must be fulfilled) are:

• i) Total QRS duration is 0.12 sec (3 small squares) or more

• ii) There is a secondary R wave in V_1 (rSr')

There is usually some secondary S–T depression and T wave inversion in the right precordial leads.

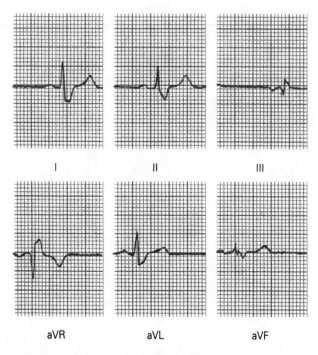

I II III

aVR aVL aVF

Complete right bundle branch block

The rhythm is sinus. The QRS complexes are broad and there is a secondary r wave in V_1. There is therefore RBBB. As is usually the case, there is a broad slurred s wave in V_6 (and is often the case also in I and aVL) and there are non-specific S–T, T changes in V_1 (often present in V_1–V_3).

126

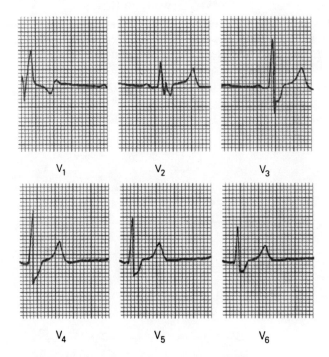

V_1 V_2 V_3

V_4 V_5 V_6

Incomplete RBBB and incomplete LBBB

The terms incomplete RBBB and incomplete LBBB are
probably best avoided. They refer to the presence of an rSr'
without a prolonged QRS (incomplete RBBB) and an R or Rs
in V_6, **without** a prolonged QRS (incomplete LBBB) but both
are normal appearances. The terms are therefore redundant.

Ventricular pre-excitation

In 1930, Wolff, Parkinson and White described a syndrome consisting of an electrocardiographic abnormality and the occurrence of episodes of paroxysmal tachycardia in otherwise healthy subjects. This syndrome now bears their names.

The ECG appearances consist of:

i) An abnormally short P–R interval (<0.10 sec).

ii) A slurring of the initial part of the QRS complex. The slurring is called the delta wave because of its resemblance to the upper case Greek letter delta (albeit one which is asymmetrically inscribed!).

iii) An increase in total QRS duration to 0.12 sec or more.

iv) Secondary S–T and T wave changes.

The ECG appearances are the result of bands of myocardium (accessory pathways) which run external to the non-conducting atrio-ventricular ring and which may lie in the left lateral area, posterior septal area, right lateral area or anterior septal area. More than one pathway may be present. In view of the fact that there are four major locations for the pathways and that one subject may have multiple pathways, the number of possible electrocardiographic appearances is large. The subdivision into types A and B is therefore no longer helpful. Now that it is possible to interrupt the pathways surgically or with radio-frequency ablation, approximate localization is of very limited value. Some idea of the localization can be obtained from the 12-lead ECG but this is a complex and uncertain procedure and it will not be attempted in detail here. Reliable detailed localizations require electrophysiological study. However, it is worth noting that the direction of the delta wave gives a clue to the accessory pathway through which conduction is occurring at the time the recording was taken. Thus a positive delta wave in V_1 indicates a **left ventricular accessory pathway** (**posteroseptal** if the delta wave and QRS are negative in II, III and aVF and **lateral** if the delta wave is isoelectric and negative in I, aVL V_5 and V_6), and a negative delta wave in V_1 indicates a **right ventricular accessory pathway** (**posteroseptal** if the delta wave and QRS are negative in II, III and aVF, situated in the right free wall if there is left axis deviation, and situated in the anteroseptal area if the axis is vertically orientated).

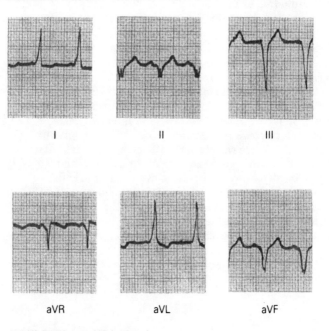

I II III

aVR aVL aVF

Wolff–Parkinson–White syndrome
- The P–R interval is short
- A delta wave is visible in I, aVL and in V_1–V_6
- The QRS is prolonged
- There are secondary S–T and T wave changes

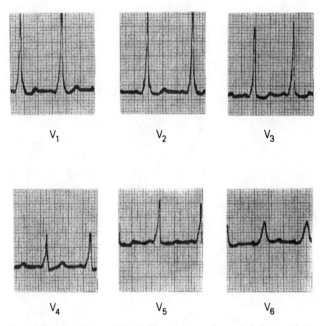

V_1 V_2 V_3

V_4 V_5 V_6

The delta wave is positive in V_1, so the pathway is left ventricular. The delta wave and QRS are negative in II, III and aVF, so the pathway is posteroseptal

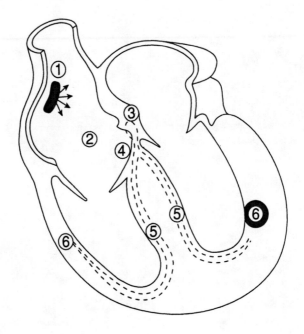

Ventricular tachycardia is caused by a rapid succession of autonomous ventricular complexes. An essential feature of ventricular tachycardia (VT) (except for the rare His bundle tachycardia) is that the QRS complexes are abnormally wide (≥ 0.12 sec) and abnormally shaped (since ventricular depolarization is initiated from an abnormal site in the ventricular myocardium). In morphology the QRS complexes of VT are similar to those in complete heart block. In rate, of course, the situation is totally different. The ventricular rate in VT may lie between 100 and 250 beats/min (typically 150–200). The rate is usually regular and the QRS shape is uniform. The appearances, therefore, are of a **broad QRS tachycardia.** Usually, there is failure of conduction retrogradely across the AV node, in which case there is no retrograde activation of the atria and normal P waves occur (at a normal rate [or possibly at a slightly increased rate as a result of baroreceptor reflex activity]). There is then atrio-ventricular dissociation again as in complete heart block but in this case, the ventricular rate is higher than the atrial rate. The recognition of occasional P waves not bearing a constant relationship to the QRS complexes and occurring at a slower rate than the QRS rate is diagnostic of VT. Fundamentally, therefore, the diagnosis of ventricular tachycardias from the 12-lead ECG ought to be straightforward — rapid, abnormally shaped and abnormally wide QRS complexes, either with no P waves visible or with P waves at a slower rate than the QRS, and not bearing a consistent relationship to the QRS complex.

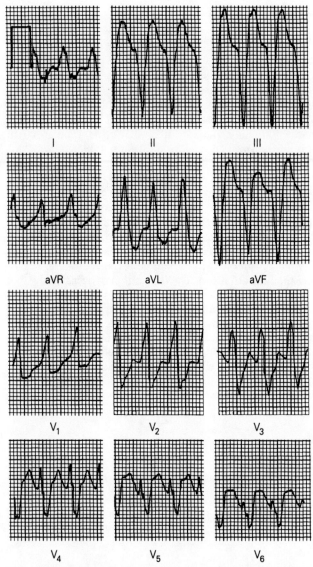

I II III

aVR aVL aVF

V_1 V_2 V_3

V_4 V_5 V_6

Broad QRS tachycardia. P wave cannot easily be identified. The third beat in V_3 looks like a fusion beat, as does the second beat in aVF. This makes the diagnosis of VT certain. The QRS in V_1 is an R wave and in V_6 is an rS complex and these features also support a diagnosis of VT

The problem is that it is possible to have a supraventricular tachycardia (SVT) with regular, abnormally wide and abnormally shaped QRS complexes in three situations:

i) supraventricular tachycardias with pre-excitation bundle branch block.

ii) supraventricular tachycardias with functional (rate-related) bundle branch block.

iii) supraventricular tachycardias with ventricular pre-excitation and antegrade conduction along the accessory pathway.

In each case, the supraventricular tachycardias could be sinus tachycardia, atrial tachycardia, atrial flutter or AVNRT. The occurrence of atrial fibrillation with pre-existing bundle branch block or with antegrade conduction along an accessory pathway probably are the mechanisms of rhythms associated with wide and **irregular** QRS complexes, often wrongly diagnosed as ventricular tachycardia. Atrial fibrillation with functional (rate-related) bundle branch block is not likely to give rise to confusion for, with the varying rates in atrial fibrillation, the degree of aberration (functional bundle branch block) will vary and the QRS complexes would have varying widths as well as varying rates.

The distinction between VT and SVT with bundle branch block or pre-excitation from the ECG is often difficult and sometimes impossible. A 12-lead record is often more helpful than a single recording and a full record should be taken wherever possible. There are some features which, when recognizable on a 12-lead record, clearly point to the diagnosis of VT in the context of a broad QRS tachycardia. These include :

i)   P waves independent of QRS complexes (ie showing a varying temporal relationship to the QRS).

ii) P wave rate recognizably less than the QRS rate.

iii) The occurrence of occasional **capture beats** (Capture beats are supraventricular (usually sinus) beats which transmit through the A-V node in the usual way and happen to reach the ventricle at a time (between the broad QRS complexes) when the ventricles are no longer refractory. A single, normal QRS complex interrupts the broad QRS tachycardias and this beat is known as a capture beat).

iv) The occurrence of occasional **fusion beats** (Fusion beats are similar to capture beats. The only difference is that the supraventricular beat travelling via the A-V node reaches the ventricles at about the same time as the next broad QRS beat of the VT and the ventricles are depolarized from two sources simultaneously, giving a fusion beat which is morphologically part way between a normal QRS and the broad QRS of VT.)

Of the above four, the finding of independent P waves is the commonest, though often none of these four diagnostic features is seen.

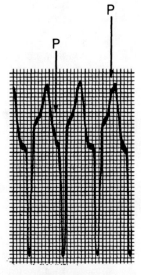

i) Independent P waves
(ie no consistent
relationship of P to QRS)

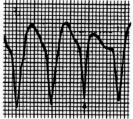

ii) Alternate QRS (only)
followed by P wave,
ie P wave rate = $\frac{1}{2}$ QRS rate

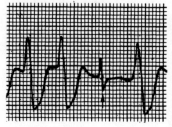

iii) Capture beat

iv) Fusion beat

137

When none of the above four diagnostic features is found, it is impossible to be **certain** of the diagnosis of VT from the 12-lead ECG (though electrophysiological studies can make the diagnosis). In that event, one has to rely on the morphology of the QRS complex to provide a guide to a **likely** diagnosis.

The main morphological features suggesting VT are as follows:

i) QRS duration ≥ 0.16 sec (when the feature is known not to be present during sinus rhythm).

ii) QRS configuration in V_1 is one of R, RS, QS, QR or Rr:

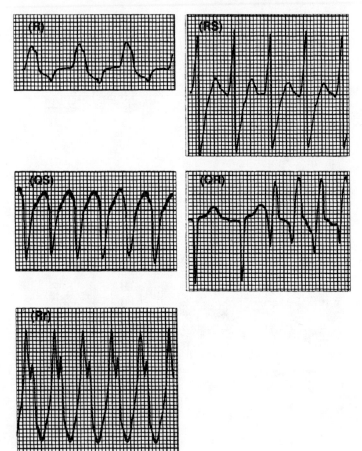

iii) QRS configuration in V_6 is one of rS, QS:
(ie r/s ratio <1)

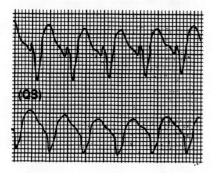

It cannot be overemphasized that the haemodynamic status of the patient is of no value in the distinction between VT and SVT. The haemodynamic status basically depends upon a combination of i) the condition of the myocardium, valves, coronary arteries and pericardium, and ii) the ventricular rate. VT should not be excluded, therefore, simply because the blood pressure and cardiac output are satisfactory.

Sometimes (as with ventricular premature beats) the abnormal QRS complexes of VT may be followed regularly by P waves (ie retrograde conduction from ventricles to atria [V–A conduction] may occur).

Ventricular extrasystoles

Ventricular extrasystoles are both premature (ie occurring earlier than would be anticipated from an inspection of preceding beats) and ectopic (ie occurring from a location other than the sino-atrial node). They are often therefore referred to as ventricular premature beats (VPBs) or ventricular ectopic beats (VEBs).

The typical appearance is of an abnormally wide ($\geq$ 0.12 sec), abnormally shaped QRS complex occurring earlier than the next scheduled normal QRS and followed by a depressed S-T segment and inverted T wave. The P wave rate is not affected since the premature ventricular depolarization does not usually travel backwards through the atrio-ventricular node. The P wave after the premature, broad QRS is not usually followed by an induced normal QRS, for the ventricles are refractory (from the VPB) when the depolarization wave reaches them. The VPB is therefore followed by a pause which is terminated when a second P wave occurs, giving rise to a further depolarization through the A–V node which then reaches a fully recovered ventricular myocardium to give a normal QRS. The time interval between the normal beat preceding and the normal beat following the VPB is exactly twice the normal sinus interval so that the pause following the VPB is said to be **compensatory.**

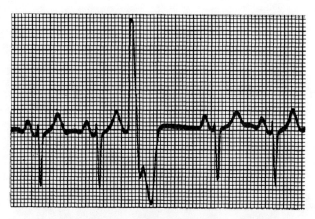

The basic rhythm is sinus tachycardia. The third beat is a
premature, broad QRS complex. It is a VPB. The third P wave can
be seen interrupting the negative T wave of the VPB. The time
interval between the second and fourth beats is exactly twice the
interval between the first and second beats. The pause between the
third and fourth beats is therefore "compensatory"

Bigeminal ventricular extrasystoles

Bigeminal ventricular extrasystoles produce a coupled rhythm; the extrasystole occurs after each contraction.
The term "trigeminal ventricular extrasystole" is occasionally used when a VPB regularly follows two sinus beats.

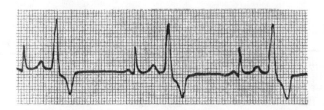

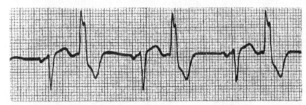

Bigeminal ventricular extrasystoles (each sinus beat is followed by a ventricular extrasystole)

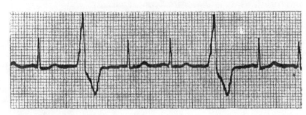

Trigeminal ventricular extrasystole

Multiple and polymorphic ventricular extrasystoles

When all VPBs have the same QRS configuration they are said to be monomorphic. When there are varying QRS waveforms the VPBs are said to be polymorphic.

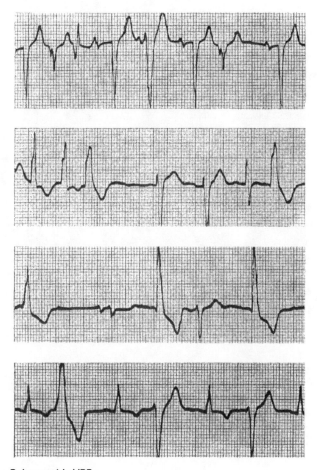

Polymorphic VPBs

Acute pericarditis

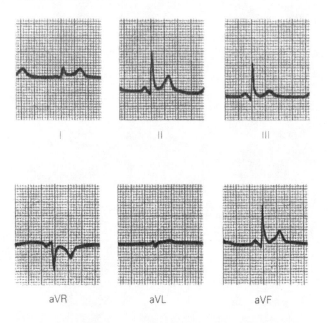

The early electrocardiographic appearance of acute (usually
viral) pericarditis is of S–T elevation concave upwards,
involving all the precordial leads and all the limb leads with a
predominantly upright QRS. In limb leads with a negative
QRS there is S–T depression and in limb leads with a very
small or equiphasic QRS the S–T segment is not obviously
deviated.

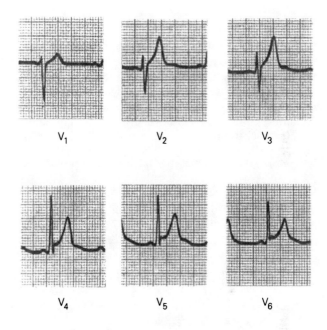

V₁ V₂ V₃

V₄ V₅ V₆

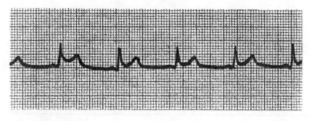

Pericarditis – initial trace. S–T elevation in I, II, III, aVF, V_1–V_6.
S–T depression in aVR

ECG in abnormal metabolic states

Metabolic disturbances have the common characteristic of disturbing the process of ventricular recovery leading to alterations of the S–T segment, the T wave and change in the duration of Q–T interval.

Hypokalaemia

The level of serum potassium causes characteristic alterations. Hypokalaemia leads to depression of the S–T segment, lowering of the T wave voltage and an increase in the size of the U wave. The U wave is a small, positive wave occurring just after the T wave. It is part of the repolarization process. The normal U wave is lower in voltage than the preceding T wave. In hypokalaemia, the U wave exceeds the T wave (which may become isoelectric) and is often mistaken for the T wave, giving rise to the belief that the Q–T interval is prolonged.

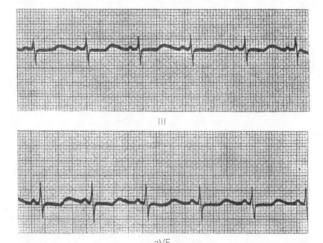

Hypokalaemia: The apparent Q–T interval is widened by increase in the duration of the T wave or, when the T wave is flattened or normal, it is followed by a very large U wave and lengthened Q–U interval.

Hyperkalaemia

This gives rise to increased length of the T waves and broadening of the QRS complexes. If the degree of hyperkalaemia increases there is progressive deterioration of intraventricular conduction and ventricular tachycardia and fibrillation ensue.

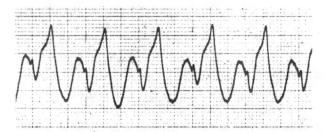

Patient in acute renal failure. Serum potassium level 8.2 mmol/l.

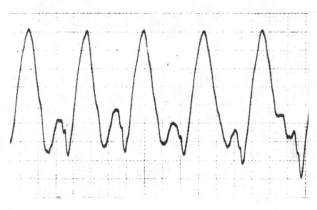

Same patient as above. Serum potassium level 9.0 mmol/l.

Action of digitalis drugs

Digitalis shortens the Q–T interval, causes a downsloping depression of the S–T segment and a reduction in the T wave height.

The rhythm is sinus. The record is normal except for the presence of S–T, T changes. There is S–T segment depression in II, III and aVF and in V_{4-6}. The T waves are of low voltage in the limb leads and in V_5 and V_6. These changes are non-specific, consistent with but not diagnostic of, digitalis effect

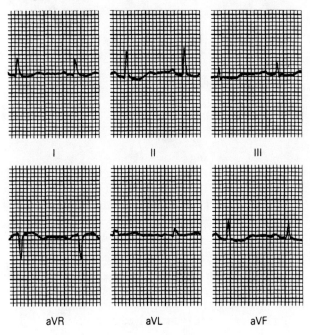

I	II	III
aVR	aVL	aVF

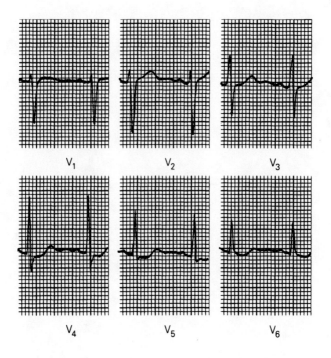

V_1 V_2 V_3

V_4 V_5 V_6

Hypothyroidism

A tracing in myxoedema is typified by sinus bradycardia, low-voltage QRS complexes, depression of the S–T segment and flattened or negative T waves in all leads.

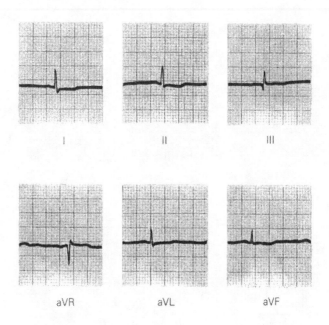

I II III

aVR aVL aVF

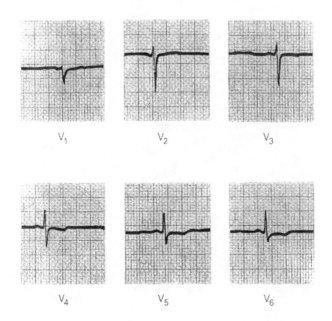

V₁   V₂   V₃

V₄   V₅   V₆

Hyperthyroidism

Hyperthyroidism gives rise to sinus tachycardia. Sometimes this might be sufficient to give a prominent atrial repolarization wave but no specific ECG changes occur.

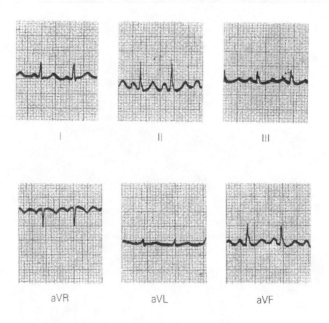

Sinus tachycardia at 130 beats/min in a female with hyperthyroidism.

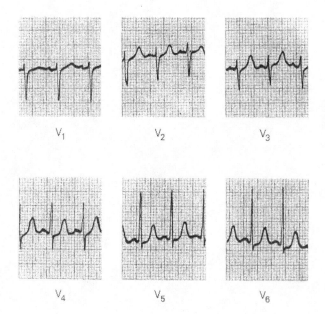

V_1 V_2 V_3

V_4 V_5 V_6

Bibliography

1. Notes on Electrocardiography. Servier Laboratories Ltd., 1971.

This small publication is based on the initial volume by BR (author's name unknown) to whom due acknowledgement is given.

2. Clinical Electrocardiography, Rowlands DJ, Gower Medical Publishing, London and New York, 1991. ISBN 0-397-44763-9.

LaVergne, TN USA
19 November 2009
164714LV00001B/126/P